Patti LaBelle's *Lite Cuisine*

Also by Patti LaBelle and Laura Randolph Lancaster

Don't Block the Blessings
LaBelle Cuisine
Patti's Pearls

Patti LaBelle

and Laura Randolph Lancaster

Patti LaBelle's

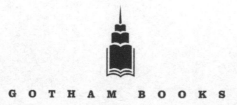

GOTHAM BOOKS

Lite Cuisine

Over 100 Dishes

With To-Die-For Taste

Made With To-Live-For Recipes

Recipe testing by David Joachim

GOTHAM BOOKS
Published by the Penguin Group
Penguin Putnam Inc., 375 Hudson Street, New York, New York 10014, U.S.A.
Penguin Books Ltd, 80 Strand, London WC2R 0RL, England
Penguin Books Australia Ltd, 250 Camberwell Road, Camberwell, Victoria 3124,
    Australia
Penguin Books Canada Ltd, 10 Alcorn Avenue, Toronto, Ontario, Canada M4V 3B2
Penguin Books (NZ) Ltd, Cnr Rosedale and Airborne Roads, Albany, Auckland 1310,
    New Zealand

Penguin Books Ltd, Registered Offices: Harmondsworth, Middlesex, England

Published by Gotham Books, a division of Penguin Putnam Inc.

First printing, April 2003

LIBRARY OF CONGRESS CATALOGING-IN-PUBLICATION DATA
LaBelle, Patti.
    Patti LaBelle's Lite Cuisine : Over 100 dishes with to-die-for taste made with
to-live-for recipes / Patti LaBelle and Laura Randolph Lancaster.
        p.   cm.
    ISBN 1-59240-004-3
    1. Cookery, American.   2. Low-fat diet—Recipes.   I. Title: Patti LaBelle's Lite
Cuisine: Over one hundred dishes with to-die-for taste made with to-live-for recipes.
II. Lancaster, Laura Randolph.   III. Title.
    TX715 .L128   2003
    641.5'638—dc21

                                                                2002155237

Printed in the United States of America

Set in Simoncini Garamond and Franklin Gothic
Designed by Judith Stagnitto Abbate / Abbate Design

Contents

Fabulous Fish *and Seafood*   35

Melt-in-Your-Mouth *Meat Dishes* 77

People-Pleasing *Poultry* 107

Scrumptious *Sides* 147

Dreamy *Desserts*   171

Acknowledgments

This book is the result of the efforts of numerous people who gave generously of their time and talent to make its publication possible. I would like to acknowledge them here for their many contributions.

Thanks to David Joachim, recipe developer and tester extraordinaire, whose talent, troubleshooting, and truly spectacular cooking skills made these recipes sing.

Thanks to the talented team at the American Dietetic Association—Jeannette F. Jordan, Registered Dietitian (RD), Certified Diabetes Educator (CDE); Jane Stephenson, RD, CED; Alison B. Evert, RD, CDE—for their informative insights and impeccable nutritional analysis. Just one question: Does the Diabetes Care and Education Practice Group of the American Dietetic Association know how lucky they are to have you three as members?

Thanks to American Dietetic Association Publisher Diana Faulhaber, who contacted, coordinated, and coolly coaxed the many comments of the ADA contributors with remarkable poise and professionalism and uncanny skill and style.

Thanks to Lori Ferme, American Dietetic Association Media Relations Manager, whose enthusiasm and excitement for this book was immediate, inspiring, and infectious.

Thanks to Rick Rodgers for just the right recommendation at just the right time.

Thanks to William R. Frederick, MD, who helped in so many ways that only he knows.

Thanks to Al Lowman for his enlightening guidance and advice.

Thanks to Carl Gullette for his heirloom photographs—and for all his help with research and remembrance.

Thanks to Patti Webster for her special and spectacular public relations skills—and her spiritual support.

Thanks to Armstead Edwards for managing the many and complex details that transform a book you have in your *head* into a book you can hold in your *hand*.

Thanks to William Shinker and the Gotham Books family for believing in this book from the start.

Thanks to Ronny B. Lancaster for opening his home, his heart—and his kitchen!—to me. But most of all for loving and supporting my sister-friend and coauthor through every phase of this book. I'm talking start to finish. Intro to ending. Deal to deadline.

And last, but by no means least, a very special and heartfelt thanks to Laura Randolph Lancaster, my coauthor and sister-friend, whose patience, professionalism, and profound gifts and talent made this book possible from concept to creation.

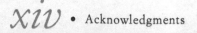

Foreword

A **few years ago,** I was preparing an invited lecture for a group of physicians on the topic of new directions in medical nutrition therapy. I had reviewed a number of recent studies that focused on comparing the effect of reduced-calorie diets with and without exercise on weight loss in obese persons. The review of these studies was not especially illuminating except for a revelation that was crystallized for me during the process: in the course of medical training, very little serious attention was paid to the appropriate use of diet therapy and exercise in the treatment of several of the worst diseases of our time—coronary heart disease, hypertension, diabetes—the list goes on and on.

And yet well over 100 million Americans are affected by these diseases, and in each case, the treatment approach begins with diet therapy and exercise. Not medication. Not surgery. Diet and exercise. This approach makes good sense because the proper use of lower-calorie diets coupled with regular programs of moderate exercise indeed results in weight loss and improvement in all of these conditions. Thus, the first line of therapy for those conditions that constitute the major epidemics of our time relates to one simple factor: *how we eat*.

The importance of a more sensible approach to our eating habits has never been more apparent in our society. We are witnessing a rise in the number of overweight and obese adults to levels of 50 percent or more. Levels of obesity in children and adolescents are also rising sharply. These statistics are particularly disturbing when you consider the long list of serious, potentially lethal, illnesses directly linked to obesity—heart disease, high blood pressure, and stroke, to name a few. Then there is diabetes. As a result of the sharply rising obesity levels, there is an explosive epidemic of type 2 diabetes. That's the bad news. The good news is that it has now been proven with an important federally funded clinical trial that even those persons who are obese and at a high risk for type 2 diabetes can prevent the development of the disease by the use of two techniques: diet therapy and exercise. Consequently, our ability to manage and to prevent some of the most damaging diseases in our society, for *all people,* depends heavily on our society taking a more balanced and sensible approach to our food choices and eating habits.

Given the short amount of time we now spend in both the preparation and consumption of meals, it is apparent that we are a society that worships at the throne of convenience. So-called "fast foods" have begun to dominate our eating habits, and because these foods tend to be high in saturated fat and in simple sugar content, when they are eaten regularly and in the portion sizes in which they are usually served, the stage is set for weight gain. Why are they so popular? Partly because they are so convenient, but also because they taste good. In fact, one of the biggest barriers to healthier eating is that most people believe that "healthy" eating must involve consumption of food that is unexciting or worse— they think it must not taste good. Enter Patti LaBelle and her cookbook *Lite Cuisine.* One of the many contributions Patti has made is to succeed in destroying such misguided perceptions. Patti understands how important healthier eating is for all of us—people with disorders like hypertension, diabetes, and atherosclerosis, people who are at risk for these problems, and people who are not at especially high risk but who simply want to pursue good health habits. But more importantly in this book, Patti LaBelle, again teaming up with Laura Randolph Lancaster, provides ample evidence that it is possible—and not very difficult— for us to enjoy healthier eating with food that is good *for* us and tastes good *to* us.

To quote one of Patti's signature songs, this is the kind of approach to eating that can lead to a "new attitude" about what it means to eat healthy. In fact, this book really highlights the notion that the presence of a disease like diabetes should not be required to force attention on healthier eating, but only the necessity for each of us to pursue better overall health. The person with diabetes and the person without any serious health issues have a similar need to pursue healthier eating. The person with diabetes or another disorder just may have a greater urgency to do so. Perhaps more important is the fact that it is not necessary to take on the frustrating challenge of "fad diets" to achieve the goal of healthier nutrition.

Patti now makes it easier for us to accomplish the important goal of healthier eating while preserving the joy that should accompany mealtimes. The recipes and offerings contained in this volume represent the kind of thoughtful attention

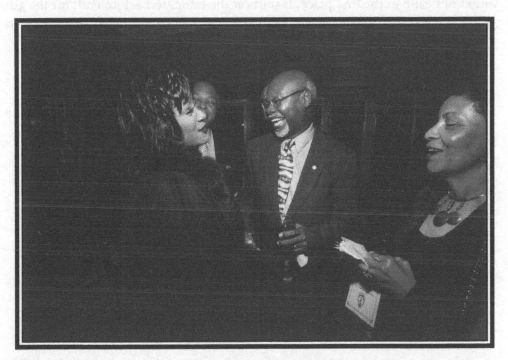

Sharing a laugh with Dr. Gavin and his lovely wife Annie after I asked him to see what he could do to get his diabetes expert friends to figure out a way to remove the carbs and sugar from my Dad's famous cinnamon rolls. Just for the record Dr. G, I wasn't kidding! (Photo by Horace Henry)

that needs to be paid to this important problem if we are to make any progress at all in our efforts to curb the explosive epidemics of obesity and diabetes in our adults and children, and if we are to reduce the devastating impact of coronary heart disease and strokes that result from atherosclerosis. The pathway to reduction of the illness and death, and the hundreds of billions of dollars in health care costs associated with all of these diseases, begins with the same step: how we eat.

This book is a celebration of good news about eating and its relationship to health. It *is* possible to eat healthier and with enjoyment. I am especially grateful to Patti for sharing her joy of food with all of us, and particularly for showing us how food that is good for us can really be good. This book deserves shelf space and regular use by all of us who are concerned not only about the improved treatment of established diseases, but also about the prevention of disease and preservation of health in the first place. It starts at the table, so I salute Patti for the gift of her insights and experiences in the kind of food preparation that will help us do all these things with joy.

James R. Gavin III, M.D., Ph.D.
Past President, American Diabetes Association
President, the Morehouse School of Medicine

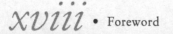

Introduction

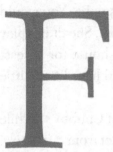**ood. How do I** love it? Let me count the ways.

And, believe me, love is the right word here. Everything about food fills me with joy—cooking it, eating it, preparing it, sharing it. I've felt that way since I was a kid. When I was a little girl growing up in Philly, hanging out in the kitchen with Chubby—that's what everybody called my mother—and her best friend, my adopted aunt Naomi, was my idea of heaven. Until I was twelve years old, in fact, the phrase "attached to your mother's apron strings" wasn't a metaphor *to* me; it was a description *of* me.

To say this caused Chubby more than a few problems would be putting it kindly. But, to her credit, my mother would let me hang out in the kitchen as long as she could stand it. Many days, however, she couldn't stand it for very long. You have to remember that, by today's standards, you would have to enlarge our kitchen just to call it small. (Can you say walk-in closet?) Even so, I'm sure Chubby and Aunt Naomi could have found a way to maneuver around it had I complied with the only thing Chubby asked me to do when they were cooking: sit still at the table. But that would be like asking me to sit still at the New Orleans jazzfest. Yeah, right. That's going to happen. Besides, whenever I was in Chubby's kitchen I was on a mission. One that in no way, shape, or form could be accomplished by sitting still at a table, or anywhere else for that matter. Whenever I was in Chubby's kitchen, I was either trying to sneak something out of whatever heavenly dish she and Aunt Naomi were cooking or trying to soak up the secrets of how they were cooking it. And even a little kid knows that to do either one right, you need a front-row seat at the stove!

When Chubby had tripped over me one too many times, she would either bribe me or threaten me ("By the time I count to three you better have your dusty little behind out of this kitchen") to get me to go outside and play with the other kids. But I never did. Even as a little kid, for me, the call of the kitchen was just too strong. Playing hide-and-seek couldn't compare with playing haute cuisine. No way, no how, no day.

Now, don't get me wrong; that doesn't mean I didn't get out of Chubby's kitchen, at least on threat days. Aunt Naomi used to say that whenever Chubby gave me The Look—the one that said, "Do-not-try-me-child-because-I-am-not-playing-with-you"—I ran out of the kitchen door so fast I left smoke. You would have, too, had you known Chubby. She was an "old school" mom. She didn't play that I-think-you-need-a-time-out stuff. If I weren't out of the house (or at least the kitchen) within ten seconds after the threat, Chubby would have lit my little behind up.

But let me get back to the kitchen—my imaginary one, not Chubby's. While all of the neighborhood kids hung out in the park across the street from our house, my refuge was the shed in the back of it. Of course, I didn't think of it as a shed. I imagined it was an internationally famous restaurant where I was an internationally famous chef. I loved spending time in that shed almost as much as I loved spending time in Chubby's kitchen. Because inside that shed I could be the person I was inside my head. And inside my head I wasn't shy little knobby-kneed Patsy Holte. I was a magnificent and multitalented (did I mention head-turning-drop-dead-fall-down-on-the-floor-and-weep gorgeous?) singing star known the world over for my meals and my music. People who had heard my singing and people who had tasted my cooking couldn't decide which was more exquisite: my four-octave range or my five-star cuisine. Ah, the power of innocence and imagination. Even now, just thinking about all the hours I spent inside that raggedy little backyard shed "cooking" all my favorite recipes gives me goose bumps.

Almost half a century later, cooking and singing still fill me with the same intense pleasure, the same immense peace. Next to singing, in fact, there is nothing I love more in this world than cooking. (Okay, so maybe I love eating a *little* more, but not much.) When I go out on tour, the first two things I pack are my hot sauce and my electric frying pans. Ask anyone who knows me: When it comes to my pans, I don't play. If my suitcases are full, I'll leave a gown or two at home before I'll walk out the door without them. That's because, in a pinch, I can usually find a fabulous outfit in whatever city I'm in without too much time or trouble. But finding a fabulous pan? Sugar, that's a whole different movie. Like I tell a couple of my in-a-hurry-to-get-married girlfriends, finding a fabulous pan is like finding a fabulous man. It takes time, honey. Time and knowledge. You shouldn't let yourself be rushed into a relationship with either. Both are just too singular, too special, too *personal*. The pan you will use to feed your stomach. And the man, well, if he's the right one, will feed your soul.

Then there's all the time you're going to be spending in one another's company—again, I'm talking about the pan and the man. More days than not you're going to be cooking up a lot of different, wonderful stuff together. Some days, hopefully most days, it's going to turn out fine. But some days it's not. Which means you need to know—not wonder, guess, or speculate but *know*—what's going to happen when (a) the fire goes out as, I promise you, even in the best of circumstances, it occasionally will, (b) your appetites aren't in synch, or (c) the mixture (either the recipe or the relationship) reaches a boiling point.

Given those realities, you have to be clear about what you're looking for—in the pan and the man. As a newly single woman starting a new life after years of living in a not-so-terrific marriage, and a newly diagnosed diabetic starting a new way of cooking after years of preparing not-so-healthy recipes, trust me when I tell you that the right one of each is the secret to happy results. Which is why it is so important to know just what you need in both. I'm talking exact qualities. Precise specifications. Specific traits. None of this roughly-speaking-more-or-less-something-sort-of-like-that kind of stuff. Clear-cut, nonnegotiable qualities. If, for example, you know you want to get involved in cooking with a minimum of fats, a good-quality nonstick pan is what you need. On that same tip, if you know you want to get involved in a relationship with a maximum of commitment, a good-quality stick-with-you man is the answer to your needs.

Once you settle on the essentials, remember this: that should be all you settle on. Or I should say that's all you should settle *for*. When it comes to the right pan and the right man, I'll sum up LaBelle's Law in four words: don't barter or bargain. Not with anything you really need. Not with anything fundamental or elemental to your dreams and desires, I don't care how glossy, gleaming, or glittery the promises or the packaging may be. After that, the rest is a cakewalk. After that, there are just two things to remember—again about the pan and the man. Both need to be able to simmer or sizzle with just the right amount of heat. And both should be super high quality without being super high maintenance.

As you can tell, I'm more than just a little passionate about my pans. (High-heel pumps have the same effect on me but that's a different story for a different book.) But it's not a fetish, at least not the way my thing for shoes is. I won't lie: I love the pumps just for the pumps. But my pan passion is different. My pan passion is a by-product of my passion for cooking. I *love* it—the shopping and the searching for just the right ingredients, the mixing and the blending of them in just the right amounts, the nothing-like-it-in-the-world thrill of a dish coming out just right.

When I wrote *LaBelle Cuisine,* my first cookbook, I realized for the first time that my cooking passion, like my pan passion, is a by-product, too. The result of one of my favorite parenting lessons: that cooking isn't just about filling people's stomachs—although, don't get me wrong, that is crucially important—but it's also about filling people's spirits. It's about bringing folks together around a table for love and laughter and camaraderie and companionship. It's about creating the roots and rhythms of our lives. There's soul food (think: grits and greens) and there's *soul* food (think: friendship and fellowship). I learned that lesson as a little kid. As an adult, I've been to enough fancy schmancy restaurants where snobby chefs thought cooking was about showing off. They couldn't be more wrong. Cooking is about showing *love.*

Cooking is the way *everyone* in my family showed love. When I was growing up, for example, every Sunday after church Chubby prepared a feast and invited the whole neighborhood. It was always an all-you-can-eat buffet. And, unlike at her Saturday night card parties, on Sundays, not only was everyone invited *to* the house, everything you ate was *on* the house. And though I know it was hard for her, after she and my father separated, Chubby let Daddy come over every weekend to make breakfast for my sisters and me. No prior arrangement necessary. No questions asked.

My father loved to cook almost as much as my mother. And, thanks to his mother, Daddy was just as good at it. My grandmother Tempie was known all over Georgia for her phenomenal cooking. Her garden was almost as famous. My aunts Hattie Mae and Joshia Mae said she grew everything in it—collards, okra, tomatoes, corn—and she'd fix baskets of her garden goodies for all her neighbors. Before she died of leukemia at the age of thirty-three, Grandmother Tempie taught Daddy all of her secret recipes. Looking back, I think that's why he loved to cook so much. I'm sure it's why he, too, subscribed to the food = love school of thought. Before he got sick, Daddy bought two restaurants and, next to his family, they were the love of his life. If you were a regular customer at either and Daddy knew your money was funny, he let you eat for free until your fortunes improved. Until Alzheimer's disease stole his mind, Daddy loved nothing better than spending all day in his restaurant cooking for his customers.

Then there are my aunts Hattie Mae and Joshia Mae. Now, I've known some people who knew their way around a kitchen, but at eightysomething, these two could teach Julia Child a thing or three about the art of fine food. Aunt Hattie and Aunt Josh invented the food = love school of thought. They put the "comfort" in comfort food. If a friend or neighbor gets sick, they go into hyper cooking made. Between the two of them, they will feed your family, your friends, and *their* family and friends for a month. I could go on and on but you get the point.

So why am I telling you all of this? Especially since, if you read my first cookbook, you've heard some of it before. So you can understand how central, how significant, how *special* a role food has always played in my life. It's this history, this lifelong love affair with food, that sent me into denial—and then into depression—when I learned I had diabetes. I just couldn't handle it, at least not at first. When I found out I had diabetes, I felt like part of my world—one of the best parts—was ending. And I wasn't even close to being ready to let it go. "The torch of love is lit in the kitchen," Aunt Naomi used to say. When I learned I had diabetes, I thought I would never be able to light it again.

And there was something else that made the news so hard to take. When it came to diabetes, I was carrying around some heavy emotional baggage. Diabetes killed Chubby. Diabetes took my mother away from this world before her time. But first it took a heartbreaking toll on her—and on me. Several years before Chubby died, I had to do something beyond disturbing, beyond disheartening, beyond difficult. Something that still haunts me. I had to give Chubby's doctors permission to amputate both her legs. It was, they said, the only way to save her. And while I know they were right, I also know this: when they took Chubby's legs, they took part of *her*. Her strength. Her spunk. Her spirit.

As painful as those memories are, in their own way, they have also been a blessing. Because remembering the toll diabetes took on my mother made me get real about taking care of myself. After several difficult months, months in which I threw myself what my sister-friend, Cassie, refers to as "the Patti pity party," I stopped crying about what I *didn't* have and started thinking about what I *did*. And what I had was a pretty terrific life. What I had was more time in this world than any of my three sisters ever got. Not one of them lived to see her forty-fourth birthday. Not Vivian. Not Barbara. Not Jackie. Cancer took them away when they were young and beautiful and in the prime of their lives.

Then there was Llona Gullette. Llona was my homegirl. She doesn't know it, but she helped me get over my depression over having diabetes, too. Llona and I went all the way back to junior high school together. The two of us practically grew up in each other's houses and I knew there was nothing in this world she wouldn't do for me. Llona had such a special place in my heart because she was my friend when I was Patsy Holte. That's who she loved—not Patti LaBelle. Like my sisters, Llona fought as long as she could but I lost her to cancer two years ago, at the age of fifty-seven.

It's the passing of so many people I loved so much, so many people who would have given anything for a diagnosis like mine, that snapped me out of the Patti pity party. Thinking about what they went through made me stop focusing on the bad news (diabetes is a chronic condition that has no cure) and start focusing on the good news (while no one can cure it, I could manage it—and lead a full and active life in the process).

That's when I decided *LaBelle Cuisine* deserved a sequel. Because that's when I decided to take the first—and most important step—in controlling my diabetes: changing the way I ate. And that meant changing the way I cooked. Not just because of the ingredients I was accustomed to using (butter, sugar, cream) and the quantities in which I used them (loads, lots, loads more). That was only half of the reason. The other half was that I cannot stomach boring, bland, bad-tasting food. When it comes to taste, I'm a rice pudding, not a rice cake, kind of girl.

Given that fact, I knew that if I wanted to eat healthier, at least in any serious, long-term way, I had to come up with recipes that were as good *to* me as they were good *for* me. And so I started talking to health and nutrition experts about healthier cooking. Why it was important. How to go about it. Who needed to do it. It was what they told me about who needed to do it that knocked me for a loop. Without dispute, without disagreement, without exception, they all agree: the way we eat is central to the health and well-being of *every single one of us*. Not just diabetics. Not just overweight people. Everybody. That's because what we eat determines what we weigh. And what we weigh determines our risk for all kinds of serious, potentially deadly, diseases. High blood pressure, heart disease, diabetes, strokes—these and other serious diseases are linked directly to obesity. And millions of people in this country are obese. Millions more are overweight. And experts say if we keep putting on weight at the current rate, almost everyone in the country is going to be overweight by 2030. That is just so deep.

That's why this is not a diabetic cookbook. Nor is it a *diet* cookbook. I spent far too many years of my life going on all kinds of crazy fad diets so I could look like one of those skinny little nineteen-year-olds they put on magazine covers. I was a grown woman in my forties before I realized that, when it comes to beauty, *one size fits all*. So while it's important to be fit (read: a healthy weight for your age and size), it's equally important to remember that Barbie is a doll, not a goal.

I know what you're thinking: if it's not a diabetic cookbook and it's not a diet cookbook, what kind of cookbook *is* it? A cookbook for people who, like me, want to eat healthier food that tastes great. A cookbook that offers lighter versions of the kind of food we all love to eat. A cookbook that I hope reflects the wise advice I heard as a kid but didn't appreciate until I was an adult: treat your body like a temple, not an amusement park.

While we all need to heed that advice, if there's one thing I've learned while writing this book it's this: unlike beauty, when it comes to nutritional needs and calorie requirements there's no such thing as one size fits all. Which means that every recipe is not going to fit every reader's needs. Every recipe does, however, include nutritional analysis, diabetic exchanges, and carbohydrate choices. With this information, information calculated by a team of nutrition experts at the American Dietetic Association, each person can "make responsible eating choices that serve their body temple." (I heard a registered dietician say that; don't you just love it?) Let's say, for example, that you're trying to shake the salt habit. You can omit it from the recipe or vary the amount to suit your needs. Or let's say you're counting carbohydrates. If you plan to have dessert at dinner, you're going to have to pass on the pasta and the potatoes.

According to the American Dietetic Association, the nation's largest organization of food and nutrition professionals, a healthy daily meal plan includes at least:

- 3 servings of vegetables
- 2 servings of fruit
- 6 servings of grains, beans, and starchy vegetables
- 2 servings of low-fat or fat-free milk
- about 6 ounces of meat or meat substitute
- small amounts of fat and sugar

The actual amounts will depend on the number of calories you need, which in turn depends on your size, age, and activity level. You should consult a registered dietician or your physician to determine your personal nutrition needs.

On a similar note, I need to say a quick word about how the nutritional analysis was calculated. When a choice of ingredients is given, the first ingredient listed is the one calculated in the analysis. Only the amount of marinade that is absorbed during preparation is calculated. And options are not included in the per serving information or the nutritional analysis.

Now that we've gotten all that straight, it's time to do some cooking *new millennium* Patti-style.

Stunningly Delicious

Salads, Soups,

and Sandwiches

Out-of-This-World Watercress Salad
with Balsamic Vinaigrette Dressing

Thanks to bagged watercress, putting this salad together doesn't get any easier. When you're preparing it, remember that watercress is very perishable, so try and buy it the same day you're planning to serve this salad.

Makes 12 servings

BALSAMIC VINAIGRETTE

½ cup extra-virgin olive oil
¼ cup balsamic vinegar
2 tablespoons chopped fresh basil
2 tablespoons chopped fresh chives
1 tablespoon minced shallots
1 teaspoon Dijon mustard
1 garlic clove, minced
¼ teaspoon salt
⅛ teaspoon white or black pepper

WATERCRESS SALAD

1 pound watercress, tough stems trimmed
2 large red tomatoes, cut into bite-size wedges
1 large yellow tomato, cut into bite-size wedges
1 sweet onion, such as Vidalia, thinly sliced
1 large cucumber, peeled, quartered lengthwise, and sliced
1 red bell pepper, seeded and cut into short strips
1 cup radishes, cut into bite-size pieces
½ cup fresh mushrooms, quartered
½ cup hearts of palm, cut into bite-size pieces

To make the vinaigrette: Combine the oil, vinegar, basil, chives, shallots, mustard, garlic, salt, and pepper in a container with a tightly sealed top (a small canning jar works well). Cover tightly and shake well, until dressing is well blended. Use immediately or refrigerate, covered, until ready to use. Shake well before serving.

To make the watercress salad: In a large bowl, toss the watercress, red tomatoes, yellow tomato, onion, cucumber, bell pepper, radishes, mushrooms, and hearts of palm. Drizzle with the vinaigrette and toss to coat.

Patti's Pointers: I like to buy bagged watercress because it's triple-washed and nearly ready to serve. Look for it near the herbs or lettuces in most supermarkets. I like to *eat* watercress because it has a delicate peppery taste—a refreshing change from plain ol' iceberg lettuce. To trim, tear off (or cut off) any thick, tough stems. But leave the smaller stems intact. They add crunch to the salad. Look for hearts of palm in the canned vegetable aisle of the supermarket. They are the tender "heart" of the tropical cabbage palm tree and taste a bit like an artichoke heart. If you can't find hearts of palm, you can use chopped artichoke hearts instead.

Per Serving: 110 calories, 2 g protein, 5 g carbohydrate, 10 g fat, 1.5 g saturated fat, 0 mg cholesterol, 1 g dietary fiber, 105 mg sodium

Diet Exchanges: 1 vegetable, 2 fats, or 0 carbohydrate choices

Sensational Salad Niçoise

This recipe is full of so many great ingredients it's not a side salad, Sugar, it's a meal. When serving Salad Niçoise, I know most people like to arrange all the different ingredients in separate little piles. Me? I like to put mine in a big bowl and toss them all together. If you're a spicy food lover like me, here's a great trick to try: swap the Niçoise olives for one 2.25-ounce can of well-drained sliced black olives—with jalapeño. Yum!

Makes 6 servings

DRESSING

¼ cup chopped shallots
⅓ cup low-sodium chicken broth
2 tablespoons olive oil
2 tablespoons fresh lemon juice
1 tablespoon white wine vinegar
1 teaspoon Dijon mustard
1 tablespoon fresh chopped basil or ½ teaspoon dried
1 tablespoon fresh chopped oregano or ½ teaspoon dried
¼ teaspoon salt
¼ teaspoon freshly ground black pepper
¼ teaspoon hot pepper sauce
⅛ teaspoon red pepper flakes

SALAD

6 ounces thin French green beans (haricots verts) or regular green beans, trimmed
8 ounces small red potatoes, thinly sliced, skin left on
One 12-ounce can reduced-sodium white tuna packed in water, drained and
  flaked
½ small red onion, halved and thinly sliced
1 cucumber, peeled, seeded, and chopped
1 pint cherry tomatoes, halved, or 1 pint grape tomatoes, left whole
½ cup Niçoise olives
1 head romaine lettuce, torn into leaves
2 large hard-cooked eggs, each peeled and cut into quarters

To make the dressing: Mix the shallots, broth, oil, lemon juice, vinegar, mustard, basil, oregano, salt, black pepper, hot pepper sauce, and red pepper flakes in a 2-cup jar or bowl. Cover and shake or whisk (if using a bowl) until well mixed. Refrigerate until the salad is ready.

Bring two pots of water to a boil. In one, cook the green beans until crisp-tender, about 5 minutes. In the other, cook the potatoes, covered, until tender, 8 to 10 minutes. Drain the beans and potatoes and run under cold water until cooled. Transfer to a large bowl.

Add the tuna, onion, cucumber, tomatoes, and olives to the bowl. Drizzle the dressing evenly over the salad. Using your hands or two large spoons, gently toss the salad to coat. Refrigerate for 1 hour.

Before serving, bring to room temperature and serve over lettuce leaves garnished with the egg quarters.

Patti's Pointers: If your market carries seedless English cucumbers, buy that instead of a regular cucumber. No seeding required! And English cucumbers tend to be less bitter than regular cucumbers. You'll need 1½ to 2 cups chopped.

Also: To trim the green beans quickly, line up all the ends on a cutting board (as many as will fit on your board!) then make a single cut across the ends with a large knife. And last but not least, to make perfect hard-cooked eggs, place the eggs in a single layer in a small saucepan and cover with cold water by 1 inch. Bring to a boil over high heat. Just when the water boils, remove the pan from the heat, cover, and let sit for 15 minutes. Drain and run cold water over the eggs until cooled. Let sit in cold water until completely cooled.

Per Serving: 240 calories, 19 g protein, 17 g carbohydrate, 11 g fat, 2 g saturated fat, 95 mg cholesterol, 4 g dietary fiber, 640 mg sodium

Diet Exchanges: 3 meats, 2 fats, 1 starch, or 1 carbohydrate choice

Cajun Chicken Caesar Salad

Makes 6 servings

CHICKEN

1 tablespoon Cajun seasoning
1 teaspoon poultry seasoning
Four 6-ounce boneless, skinless chicken breast halves

SALAD

3 tablespoons extra-virgin olive oil
3 tablespoons fresh lemon juice
2 tablespoons reduced-sodium chicken broth or water
2 tablespoons reduced-fat sour cream
1 teaspoon Dijon mustard
¾ teaspoon red pepper sauce, such as Tabasco
2 tablespoons grated Parmesan cheese
1 head romaine lettuce

To make the chicken: Preheat the oven to 375°F. Coat a baking sheet with fat-free cooking spray.

In a small bowl, mix together the Cajun seasoning and poultry seasoning. Sprinkle evenly over both sides of the chicken breasts.

Place on the prepared baking sheet and bake until an instant-read thermometer registers 160°F in a breast and juices run clear, about 25 to 30 minutes.

To make the salad: In a large bowl, combine the oil, lemon juice, broth or water, sour cream, mustard, red pepper sauce, and Parmesan.

Tear the lettuce into large leaves and toss with the dressing to coat evenly.

Divide the lettuce among 6 salad plates. Slice the chicken into strips and divide among the plates.

Option: This dish tastes great as a wrap sandwich (even the next day!). Heat up some of the chicken strips and a large tortilla in the microwave oven, about 30 seconds. Then roll up with the dressed romaine lettuce.

Per Serving: 190 calories, 24 g protein, 3 g carbohydrate, 9 g fat, 2 g saturated fat, 60 mg cholesterol, less than 1 g dietary fiber, 370 mg sodium

Diet Exchanges: 3 very lean meats, 1½ fats, or 0 carbohydrate choices

Luscious Lobster Salad

Make sure you refrigerate this dish at least four hours before serving—longer if you have the time. That way the flavors can really come together and develop. If you cover tightly and refrigerate it overnight, you'll have a seriously *great* salad, not just a seriously *good* one. And for the price of lobster tails these days—I almost fainted the last time I bought some!—great is exactly what this salad should be.

Makes 4 servings

⅓ cup reduced-fat mayonnaise, such as Hellmann's Just 2 Good!
2 teaspoons fresh lemon juice
1 teaspoon Dijon mustard
1 teaspoon extra-virgin olive oil
1 tablespoon chopped fresh tarragon
¼ teaspoon salt
¼ teaspoon ground black pepper
⅛ teaspoon ground red pepper
⅛ teaspoon paprika
2 lobster tails, thawed if frozen (about 1 pound total)
4 cups arugula or other lettuce leaves
1 tomato, cut into 8 wedges

In a medium bowl, combine the mayonnaise, lemon juice, mustard, olive oil, tarragon, salt, black pepper, red pepper, and paprika.

Bring a pot of lightly salted water to boil. Boil the lobster tails until just firm and opaque throughout, 8 to 9 minutes.

Drain and rinse the tails under cold water (it's easiest to do this with tongs). Cut each tail in half lengthwise right through the shell (if the meat is not opaque all the way through, boil the halved shells for another minute or so).

Scoop the lobster meat from the shells with your fingers. Cut into bite-size pieces (you should have about 2 cups lobster meat). Gently fold the lobster meat into the mayonnaise mixture. Cover and refrigerate for at least four hours, preferably overnight.

Put the arugula or other lettuce on a platter or plates. Top with the lobster salad and garnish with the tomato wedges.

Patti's Pointers: It's easier to cut the lobster tails if they don't curl up during cooking. To keep the tails from curling as they cook, skewer them lengthwise with short metal or bamboo skewers. I use arugula in this recipe because its peppery bite is the perfect complement to this mild and creamy lobster salad. But if you don't like the taste, try romaine lettuce instead. It has six times as much vitamin C and up to ten times as much beta-carotene as iceberg lettuce. Just remember: generally speaking, the greener the lettuce leaves, the more nutrition they contain.

Per Serving: 150 calories, 14 g protein, 6 g carbohydrate, 7 g fat, 3 g saturated fat, 60 mg cholesterol, less than 1 g dietary fiber, 650 mg sodium

Diet Exchanges: 2 meats, 1 fat, or ½ carbohydrate choice

Crab Louis

Makes 8 servings

1 cup reduced-fat mayonnaise, such as Hellmann's Just 2 Good!
½ cup chili sauce
¼ cup finely chopped red pepper
¼ cup finely chopped green onions
1½ teaspoons prepared horseradish
¼ teaspoon salt
¼ teaspoon red pepper flakes
1 head iceberg lettuce, shredded (about 8 cups)
1 pint cherry or grape tomatoes
2 pounds fresh jumbo lump crabmeat, picked over to remove shells

In a large bowl, mix together the mayonnaise, chili sauce, red pepper, green onions, horseradish, salt, and red pepper.

Arrange the shredded lettuce on a platter and decorate the edge of the platter with the tomatoes. Gently scoop the crabmeat on top of the lettuce, being careful not to break up the lumps. Spoon ½ cup of the dressing over the crabmeat. Serve the remaining dressing in a small bowl.

Patti's Pointers: You can make this dish ahead of time, then assemble just before serving. Refrigerate the dressing for up to 2 days. Prepare the platter of lettuce and tomatoes, cover, and refrigerate for up to 1 day. Then simply top with the crab and dressing, and you're good to go.

Per Serving: 290 calories, 37 g protein, 10 g carbohydrate, 10 g fat, 1.5 g saturated fat, 170 mg cholesterol, less than 1 g dietary fiber, 880 mg sodium

Diet Exchanges: 3 meats, 1½ fats, 2 vegetables, or ½ carbohydrate choice

Berry Cool Chicken Chili

I got this recipe from one of the most gorgeous and talented women on the planet—Halle Berry. You know that commercial where the model says, "Don't hate me because I'm beautiful"? Well, I won't lie: If the child weren't so sweet, I

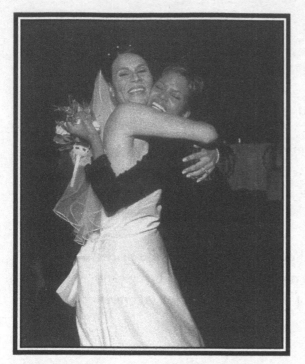

Halle-lujah! That's what I said when Girlfriend caught the bouquet at the wedding of my co-author and sister-friend, Laura Randolph Lancaster. (Photo by Roosevelt Sharpe)

would have to hate her. But I can't. She's as beautiful on the inside as she is on the outside, and when you've got a face and body like hers, that is saying something, right? The night she won the Academy Award for best actress, you would have thought I had won a Grammy Award for best album (Note to the Recording Academy: yes, that is a hint). When they announced Girlfriend's name on that stage, I was so happy for her I started screaming and shouting so loud I woke the whole neighborhood up. But it was her acceptance speech that had me crying like a baby. It was just like her—beautiful and gracious and real.

While everybody knows Halle is as talented as she is gorgeous, here's something you may not know about her: she's diabetic. She found out several years ago when she went into a diabetic coma on the set of her first TV show, the long-canceled sitcom *Living Dolls*. Like millions of people, Halle didn't know she had the disease. Which is why it is so important for all of us to ask our doctors about getting tested for it. When you make Halle's fabulous chili, why don't you make an appointment to do just that? Halle would like that. And so would I.

1 teaspoon olive oil
1 cup chopped onion
1 cup chopped green bell pepper
¾ cup chopped carrots
3 garlic cloves, minced
2 pounds ground chicken
1 tablespoon chili powder
1½ teaspoons dried oregano
1½ teaspoons dried basil
½ teaspoon ground cumin
½ teaspoon salt
½ teaspoon red pepper flakes
One 14.5-ounce can no-salt-added diced tomatoes, undrained
One 15-ounce can great northern beans, rinsed and drained
One 14.5-ounce can fat-free reduced-sodium chicken broth
One 6-ounce can low-sodium tomato paste

Coat a large soup pot with fat-free cooking spray and add the oil. Heat over medium heat until the oil is hot. Add the onion, bell pepper, carrots, and garlic. Cook, stirring occasionally, until the vegetables are just tender, 6 to 8 minutes. Add the chicken and, breaking up the meat with a spoon, cook until the chicken is no longer pink, about 10 minutes. Pour off any fat.

Stir in the chili powder, oregano, basil, cumin, salt, and red pepper flakes. Cook about 2 minutes.

Stir in the tomatoes, beans, broth, and tomato paste. Bring to a boil over high heat. Reduce the heat to low and cook, uncovered and stirring occasionally, until the flavors come together, about 45 minutes.

Per Serving: 250 calories, 31 g protein, 23 g carbohydrate, 4 g fat, 1 g saturated fat, 65 mg cholesterol, 5 g dietary fiber, 350 mg sodium

Diet Exchanges: 3 very lean meats, 2 vegetables, 1 starch, 1 fat, or 1 carbohydrate choice

Luther's Italian Chicken Soup

You know who gave me this fabulous recipe? The one and only velvet-voiced Luther Vandross. I love Luther; he and I go way back. And when I say way back, I mean waaaaay back. Back in the sixties, when he was just a kid, Luther used to cut school to come to the Apollo Theater to see Patti LaBelle and The Bluebelles. But seeing us wasn't enough for Luther. He wanted to *meet* us. So badly, in fact, that he concocted this ingenious plan to get backstage. Luther told Peter Long, the Apollo's public relations director at the time, that he was writing a school report on The Bluebelles and if he didn't get an interview with us he would flunk. Even back then, Luther was so smooth and charming and convincing that Peter bought the story hook, line, and sinker. While I was running an errand at the time, Luther got his interview with Sarah and Nona. Even then he had chutzpa.

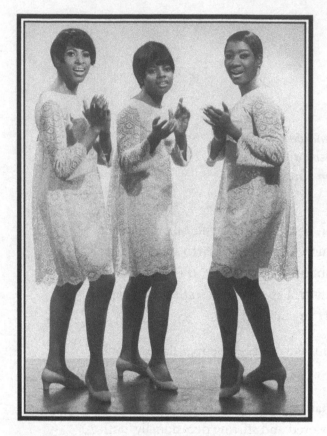

The way Nona Hendryx, Sarah Dash, and I looked when Luther used to sneak into the world-famous Apollo to see us. Check out the outfits; you couldn't tell us we weren't too cute!

Not long after the interview, Luther and his friend choreographer Bruce Wallace started the first Patti LaBelle and The Bluebelles Fan Club. Bruce was the first president, with Luther serving as his vice president. Of course, these days I'm the (unofficial) president of the Luther Vandross Fan Club. Boyfriend can sing. A voice like Luther's—silken, sexy, smooth—doesn't come along often, as evidenced by all of his hits (too many to count) and awards (Do you store them in a warehouse, honey?). Not only can he sing, but as anyone who has ever seen

Luther perform can tell you, Boyfriend can work a stage. What you may not know is that he can also work a stove. Since he learned he was diabetic, however, Luther has been into healthier cooking and eating. But don't take my word for it. Try Luther's Italian chicken soup recipe. When you taste it, you'll be singing his praises.

Makes 6 servings

1 teaspoon olive oil
1 small onion, finely chopped
½ cup chopped celery
3 garlic cloves, minced
1 pound ground chicken
Two 14.5-ounce cans no-salt-added stewed tomatoes, undrained
One 14.5-ounce can reduced-sodium fat-free chicken broth
One 8-ounce can no-salt-added tomato sauce
One 4-ounce jar chopped or sliced pimientos, drained
½ teaspoon dried Italian seasoning
½ teaspoon dried basil
½ teaspoon dried oregano
½ teaspoon salt
½ teaspoon freshly ground black pepper
1 cup uncooked rotini pasta

Coat a large soup pot with fat-free cooking spray and add olive oil. Heat over medium heat until the oil is hot. Add the onion, celery, and garlic. Cook, stirring frequently, until the vegetables are just tender, about 4 minutes. Add the chicken and cook, breaking up the meat with a spoon, until the chicken is no longer pink, about 10 minutes. Pour off any fat.

Stir in the stewed tomatoes, broth, tomato sauce, pimientos, Italian seasoning, basil, oregano, salt, and pepper. Bring to a boil over high heat. Add the pasta and return to a boil. Reduce the heat to medium-low, cover, and cook until the pasta is just tender, about 15 minutes.

Patti's Pointers: When Luther makes his delicious Italian chicken soup, he uses rotini, but I make it with stelline because it means "star"—like the super-talented one he is.

Per Serving: 250 calories, 24 g protein, 27 g carbohydrate, 6 g fat, 1.5 g saturated fat, 50 mg cholesterol, 3 g dietary fiber, 850 mg sodium

Diet Exchanges: 1 starch, 2½ very lean meat, 2 vegetables, 1 fat, or 2 carbohydrate choices

Better than Mom's Beef Stew

A delicious and complete meal in a bowl! Like most stews, this one tastes even better the next day when the flavors have had plenty of time to get to know one another. In fact, this is the kind of dish you could let sit on low heat all day, go out shoe shopping, and, come dinnertime, it would be as fierce as your new pumps.

Makes 6 servings

1 pound beef top round, trimmed of fat and cut into bite-size pieces
2 tablespoons Worcestershire sauce
One 14-ounce can fat-free reduced-sodium beef broth
One 14-ounce can Italian-style chopped fresh tomatoes, undrained
1 tablespoon prepared horseradish
2 garlic cloves, minced
1 teaspoon chili powder
½ teaspoon salt
¼ teaspoon ground black pepper
5 medium red potatoes, scrubbed and cubed
1 large onion, coarsely chopped
1 cup baby carrots, halved if large
2 ribs celery, sliced
1 tablespoon chopped fresh oregano or ½ teaspoon dried

Put the beef and Worcestershire sauce in a resealable plastic bag and shake to coat. Marinate in the refrigerator for at least 2 hours and up to 4 hours.

Coat a large saucepan or stew pot with fat-free cooking spray and heat over medium-high heat until smoking hot. Remove the beef from the marinade and add to the pan, cooking until browned all over, about 5 minutes.

Reduce the heat to low and stir in the broth, tomatoes, horseradish, garlic, chili powder, salt, pepper, and any leftover marinade. Cover and cook for 1 hour and 45 minutes. Add the potatoes, onion, carrots, celery, and oregano. Cook, covered, until the vegetables are tender, about 1 hour more. If the liquid in the pan is too thin, raise the heat to medium-high and boil until the liquid thickens.

Patti's Pointers: If you can't find beef top round, extra-lean stew beef works just as well and is up to 97 percent lean.

Per Serving: 250 calories, 23 g protein, 32 g carbohydrate, 3.5 g fat, 1.5 g saturated fat, 45 mg cholesterol, 4 g dietary fiber, 400 mg sodium

Diet Exchanges: 2 very lean meats, 2 starches, 1 vegetable, or 2 carbohydrate choices

Daniel's Chilled Spring Carrot Soup
with Lobster and Lime

You are going to fall in love with this soup recipe! It was created by the renowned French chef-restaurateur Daniel Boulud, who gave it to me when I told him I was writing *Lite Cuisine.* And when I say renowned, I mean renowned. Not only has Daniel been named chef of the year by *Bon Appetit* magazine, Boyfriend's restaurant received *Gourmet* magazine's Top Table Award. A few months ago, when the New York Public Library held its "Preserve the Cookbook Collection" benefit gala, guess where they held it? At Boyfriend's restaurant, DANIEL. The menu, by some of New York's most famous chefs, was off the hook. I'm talking seriously scrumptious. Mad fabulous. To-die-for delicious. But like I told Daniel, for $750 a plate it better be! Proceeds from the dinner benefited the cookbook collection of the New York Public Library, which is why I agreed to sing at the dinner. (You people took that "sing for your supper" saying seriously, huh?) That, and to get to sample some more of Daniel's cooking. The library has thousands of cookbooks from around the world. (Note to the staff: I will be dropping by to make sure at least two of them are by Patti LaBelle.) When Daniel makes this soup at his restaurant he uses chicken stock and heavy cream, but I lightened it up with low-sodium chicken broth and fat-free half-and-half. It's the perfect first course for your next puttin'-on-the-ritz affair.

1 tablespoon extra-virgin olive oil
1 medium leek (white part only), thinly sliced, rinsed, and patted dry
1 small onion, thinly sliced
1 rib celery, thinly sliced
1 garlic clove, peeled and left whole
6 sprigs cilantro, stems and leaves separated, leaves finely chopped
2 sprigs thyme
15 California spring carrots, peeled and thinly sliced
½ teaspoon salt
¼ teaspoon freshly ground black pepper
Pinch of sugar
5 cups fat-free, low-sodium chicken broth
3 cups fresh carrot juice
1 lime
Tabasco sauce
½ cup fat-free half-and-half
2 large lobster tails, thawed if frozen (about 1¼ pounds total)

Warm the olive oil in a medium pot over medium-low heat. Add the leek, onion, celery, and garlic. Lower the heat to medium-low and cook, stirring frequently until the vegetables are translucent but not browned, about 10 minutes. Tie together the cilantro stems and thyme sprigs with kitchen twine and add the bundle to the pot. Stir in the carrots, salt, pepper, and sugar. Cook, stirring occasionally, for 10 to 15 minutes.

Pour in the chicken broth and bring to a boil over high heat. Lower the heat to medium and simmer, skimming the surface regularly to remove any fat and foam, until the carrots are very tender, about 20 minutes. Discard the garlic clove and herb sprigs. Transfer the soup to a blender or food processor and puree until smooth (in batches if necessary). Strain the pureed soup through a fine-mesh sieve, pressing out as much liquid as possible. Cover and refrigerate the soup base until well chilled.

Once the soup base is cold, stir in the carrot juice. Finely grate the zest from the lime and set aside. Cut the lime in half and squeeze the juice from one half into the soup. (Save the other half for another use.) Stir in a few drops of Tabasco sauce. Cover and refrigerate until ready to serve.

Bring a pot of lightly salted water to boil. Add the lobster tails and boil until just firm and opaque throughout, 8 to 9 minutes. Drain and rinse the tails under cold water (it's easiest to do this with tongs). Cut each tail in half lengthwise right through the shell (if the meat is not opaque all the way through, boil the halved shells for another minute or so).

Scoop the lobster meat from the shells with your fingers. Cut into ½-inch chunks. In a medium bowl, add the chopped cilantro to the half-and-half and set aside. To serve: ladle the soup into shallow soup bowls and swirl some of the half-and-half mixture into each serving. Place some lobster chunks in the center and sprinkle with the reserved zest.

Patti's Pointers: If you don't have a juicer or can't buy fresh carrot juice at a local juice bar, use canned carrot juice instead. You'll find it near the tomato juice in most supermarkets. And let me tell you about the leeks: They are the queens of the allium world. More subtle than onion, more refined than shallots, leeks have a sweetly gentle onion flavor that is perfect for delicate soups. That's the good news. The bad news is that they also have a tendency to harbor grit in their layers. And I don't do grit. So to make sure you get all of it out, slice them first and place the slices in a bowl of water. Swish the slices around in the water, then let any dirt settle to the bottom of the bowl. Lift the leeks out with a slotted spoon and pat dry before using.

Per Serving: 110 calories, 16 g protein, 7 g carbohydrate, 2 g fat, 1 g saturated fat, 70 mg cholesterol, less than 1 g dietary fiber, 480 mg sodium

Diet Exchanges: 2 very lean meats, 1 vegetable, or ½ carbohydrate choice

Shrimp and Salmon Melts

Makes 8 servings

One 12-ounce package frozen baby shrimp, thawed
One 10-ounce can sockeye or pink salmon, packed in water, drained and flaked
¾ cup reduced-fat sour cream
¾ cup reduced-fat mayonnaise, such as Hellmann's Just 2 Good!
¼ cup finely chopped red onion
¼ cup finely chopped celery
3 tablespoons chopped fresh parsley
1 tablespoon prepared horseradish
¼ teaspoon ground black pepper
2 large beefsteak tomatoes, sliced into 8 slices each
8 English muffins, split in half
6 ounces reduced-fat sharp cheddar cheese, grated (1½ cups)

Preheat the oven to 400°F.

In a large bowl, combine the shrimp, salmon, sour cream, mayonnaise, onion, celery, parsley, horseradish, and black pepper.

Lay one tomato slice on each English muffin slice. Equally divide the seafood mixture among the English muffins. Sprinkle with the cheese.

Place in a shallow roasting pan and bake until heated through and the cheese melts, about 10 minutes.

Patti's Pointers: Not all low-fat cheeses are created equal. I like to use Cracker Barrel 2 percent sharp white cheddar cheese, which comes in block form. It melts well and has a bolder flavor than some of the milder pre-shredded varieties.

Per Serving: 290 calories, 24 g protein, 30 g carbohydrate, 7 g fat, 3 g saturated fat, 80 mg cholesterol, 2 g dietary fiber, 550 mg sodium

Diet Exchanges: 5½ meats, 2 fats, 2 starches, or 2 carbohydrate choices

Warm Tuna Wraps

This recipe takes the stress and the mess out of getting lunch on the table. Not only is it ready in a flash, it gives you all the flavor of a tuna melt with a fraction of the fat and calories.

Makes 6 servings

1½ cups frozen corn, rinsed in cold water and patted dry
One 12.5-ounce can reduced-sodium solid white tuna in water, drained and
    flaked
1½ cups reduced-fat shredded cheddar-jack cheese
¾ cup chunky salsa (you choose mild, medium, or the way I like it—hot, hot,
    hot!)
1 tablespoon chopped fresh chives or parsley (optional)
6 large (10-inch) flour tortillas

In a medium bowl, mix together the corn, tuna, cheese, salsa, and chives or parsley (if using).

Spoon one-sixth of the mixture into the middle of a tortilla. Place on a microwave-safe plate and microwave on high until heated through and cheese melts, 1 to 2 minutes. Roll the tortilla closed and serve immediately.

Per Serving: 340 calories, 31 g protein, 42 g carbohydrate, 6 g fat, 2 g saturated fat, 15 mg cholesterol, 2 g dietary fiber, 570 mg sodium

Diet Exchanges: 4 meats, 3 starches, 1 fat, or 3 carbohydrate choices

Llona's Steak Sandwiches

I can't so much as smell a cheesesteak without thinking about my homegirl, Llona Gullette. When we were teenagers, we used to eat them like they were going out of style. Philly is the home of the original cheesesteak, so the city is packed with places that sell them. When we were growing up, Llona and I always went to the same little shop to get ours—this twenty-four-hour hole-in-the-wall that made the best ones in Philly. Come to think of it, the best ones I've ever tasted *anywhere*. Sometimes, between the two of us, Llona and I only had enough money for one cheesesteak, so we'd beg the owner for extra meat and share it. Sharing was the backbone of our thirty-plus-year friendship. If I was sick, Llona would show up at my door with a bag of groceries and cook me enough meals to last a week. If I was scared or lonely, she'd stay on the phone with me until I fell asleep. When my sister Barbara got married, Llona stayed up all night helping me cook Barbara's favorite dishes for her two hundred wedding guests. And it was Llona's parents who helped my father get a job at Baldwin Locomotive when he and Chubby decided they wanted to move to Philly. Like I said, Llona and I were as close as two peas in a pod.

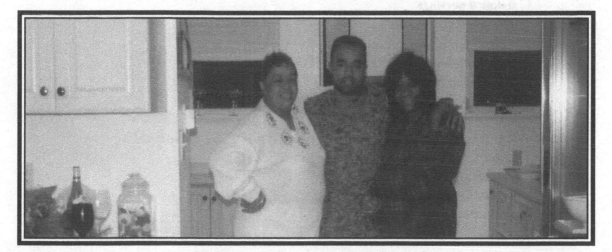

Llona, her son, Carl, and me hanging out in our favorite place—my kitchen. (Photo by Roosevelt Sharpe)

Several years ago, when Llona was diagnosed with breast cancer and called to tell me the news, I told her it was my turn to be there for her. "Anything you want, Girlfriend, just ask."

Llona hesitated. "Just one thing, Patsy," she finally said. "I want you to sing."

I didn't get it at first. "Sing?" I said. "Girl, you should be sick of hearing me sing by now. You've been to more concerts than I have."

"Not at a concert," she said quietly. "When the time comes."

We never spoke of it again. Not once. But we didn't need to. Both of us knew what had been asked—and promised.

New Year's Day, when Llona's son Carl called to tell me Llona was gone, he asked me to sing at his mother's funeral. He didn't know that if he hadn't asked me, I would have asked him.

The one thing I did ask Carl was this: "Don't list me in the program as Patti LaBelle. List me as Patsy Holte." That's who I was to Llona. That's who she loved.

At her funeral, when we sent Llona home, I sang "You Are My Friend." All I can tell you is that truer words were never spoken. Since I learned I have diabetes, my late night cheesesteak runs are a thing of the past. They were never as much fun without Llona, anyway.

Makes 4 servings

1 small red onion, sliced
⅓ cup fat-free low-sodium beef broth
½ teaspoon broiled steak seasoning, such as McCormick's
1 tablespoon steak sauce, such as A1
¼ teaspoon hot pepper sauce, such as Tabasco
¼ teaspoon freshly ground black pepper, plus more for sprinkling
12 ounces paper-thin beef round sandwich steaks
4 steak sandwich rolls, split
4 romaine lettuce leaves
1 tomato, thinly sliced

Coat a large skillet with fat-free cooking spray and heat over medium heat. Add the onions and cook until tender, about 5 minutes. Stir in the broth, steak seasoning, steak sauce, hot pepper sauce, and ¼ teaspoon of the black pepper. Bring to a boil.

Add the steak and cook, stirring frequently and separating the slices until meat is no longer pink, about 5 minutes. Sprinkle with the remaining black pepper.

Line the rolls with the lettuce and tomato slices. Spoon the steak on top and serve immediately.

Option: If you like a wet steak sandwich, top these with low-sodium tomato sauce, ketchup, or your favorite steak sauce.

Per Serving: 320 calories, 26 g protein, 38 g carbohydrate, 7 g fat, 3.5 g saturated fat, 50 mg cholesterol, 2 g dietary fiber, 520 mg sodium

Diet Exchanges: 2 medium-fat meats, 2 starches, or 2½ carbohydrate choices

Serious Sloppy Joes

These taste even better after a day or two of "marinating" in the fridge. Cover and store in the refrigerator for up to 2 days, then reheat in the microwave and serve on the buns. Be sure, however, to use regular ground turkey (which usually includes some leg meat), not 99 percent lean ground turkey *breast* meat. I won't lie: The breast meat is just too lean to make a good juicy gyro. Worse, it dries out if cooked too long.

Makes 8 servings

½ cup chopped red onion
½ cup chopped celery
3 garlic cloves, minced
1 pound 95 percent lean ground turkey (not 99 percent lean ground turkey breast)
One 8-ounce can low-sodium tomato sauce
One 6-ounce can low-sodium tomato paste
½ cup chili sauce
1 tablespoon white wine vinegar
1 teaspoon chili powder
1 teaspoon sugar substitute, such as Diabetisweet or Splenda
1 teaspoon seasoning salt, such as Lawry's
½ teaspoon ground cumin
½ teaspoon dried oregano
¼ teaspoon black pepper
8 whole-wheat hamburger buns

Coat a large skillet with fat-free cooking spray and heat over medium heat. Add the onion, celery, and garlic. Cook until just tender, about 4 minutes. Add the turkey and cook, breaking up the meat with a spoon, until the turkey is no longer pink, about 5 minutes. Drain off any excess fat.

Stir in the tomato sauce, tomato paste, chili sauce, white wine vinegar, chili powder, sugar substitute, seasoning salt, cumin, oregano, and pepper. Cover and simmer, stirring frequently, for 15 minutes to blend the flavors.

Divide the mixture equally among the hamburger buns to make sandwiches.

Per Serving: 330 calories, 19 g protein, 44 g carbohydrate, 10 g fat, 3.5 g saturated fat, 45 mg cholesterol, 4 g dietary fiber, 610 mg sodium

Diet Exchanges: 2 starches, 1 lean meat, 1 vegetable, or 3 carbohydrate choices

Lemon-Basil Chicken Pitas

Makes 2 servings

⅓ cup reduced-fat mayonnaise, such as Hellmann's Just 2 Good!
⅓ cup chopped red onion
¼ cup chopped celery
2 tablespoons chopped fresh basil
2 teaspoons fresh lemon juice
¾ teaspoon salt
⅛ teaspoon ground black pepper
One 5-ounce can chunk chicken breast in water, drained
2 cups arugula or other lettuce leaves
2 rounds pita bread, cut in half (right across the diameter of the circle)

In a medium bowl, stir together the mayonnaise, onion, celery, basil, lemon juice, salt, and pepper. Fold in the chicken, leaving as many large chunks as possible.

Divide the arugula or other lettuce among the pita halves. Spoon one-fourth of the chicken mixture into each pita half.

Patti's Pointers: If you can find small tender arugula greens at the market, buy them. Arugula has a delicious peppery bite that complements this creamy chicken salad better than plain ol' iceberg lettuce ever will. If you can't find arugula, go for romaine lettuce, which has better flavor, six times as much vitamin C, and up to ten times as much beta-carotene as iceberg lettuce.

Per Serving: 200 calories, 14 g protein, 22 g carbohydrate, 6 g fat, 1 g saturated fat, 35 mg cholesterol, 1 g dietary fiber, 730 mg sodium

Diet Exchanges: 3 very lean meats, 2 starches, 1 fat, ½ vegetable, or 1½ carbohydrate choices

Fabulous French Onion and Mushroom Turkey Burgers

Don't let the lean ground turkey fool you. When it comes to taste, these burgers give Big Macs a run for their money! ⌒⌒

Makes 4 servings

8 ounces sliced white button mushrooms
2 celery stalks, finely chopped
1 garlic clove, minced
1 egg, lightly beaten
½ teaspoon poultry seasoning
¼ teaspoon freshly ground black pepper
1 pound 95 percent lean ground turkey (not 99 percent lean ground turkey
  breast; see headnote on Serious Sloppy Joes, page 28)
1 can condensed French onion soup, such as Campbell's
4 whole-wheat hamburger buns, split in half

Coat a large skillet with fat-free cooking spray and heat over medium heat. Add the mushrooms, celery, and garlic. Cook until the mushrooms are tender, about 4 minutes. Remove from the heat and let cool.

Meanwhile, in a large bowl, stir together the egg, poultry seasoning, and black pepper. Stir in the mushroom mixture.

Using your hands, mix in the turkey, handling the meat as little as possible. Shape into 4 patties.

Add the patties to the skillet used to cook the mushrooms. Cook over medium heat until just slightly pink in the center, about 5 minutes per side. Drain off any excess fat.

Pour the soup over the burgers in the skillet (be careful, as it may spatter). Bring to a boil. Reduce the heat to low, cover, and simmer for 5 minutes. Remove the burgers and cook the remaining soup in the skillet until thickened. Serve the thickened sauce over the burgers on the buns.

Option: These burgers are plenty moist and tasty! But, if you feel the need to dress them up with something, low-fat ranch dressing makes these burgers off the hook.

Per Serving: 390 calories, 26 g protein, 42 g carbohydrate, 13 g fat, 5 g saturated fat, 120 mg cholesterol, 3 g dietary fiber, 930 mg sodium

Diet Exchanges: 2 lean meats, 2 starches, 1 fat, 1 vegetable, or 3 carbohydrate choices

Great Greek Gyros

I know most people prepare gyros with ground beef, but I use ground turkey in mine. It's the perfect alternative to ground chuck because it doesn't damage the flavor but it *does* ditch lots of the fat.

Makes 4 servings

*1 pound 95 percent lean ground turkey (not 99 percent lean ground turkey
   breast; see headnote on Serious Sloppy Joes, page 28)*
2 garlic cloves, minced
4 ounces reduced-fat feta cheese, crumbled (1 cup)
1 tablespoon chopped fresh oregano
1 teaspoon ground black pepper
4 rounds pita bread, lightly toasted
1 cup shredded lettuce
1 large tomato, thickly sliced
½ medium red onion, thinly sliced
1 cup reduced-fat sour cream

Coat a large skillet with fat-free cooking spray and heat over medium heat. Add the turkey and garlic and cook, breaking up the meat with a spoon, until the turkey is no longer pink, about 5 minutes. Drain off any excess fat.

Remove from the heat and stir in the feta, oregano, and black pepper.

Cut off about 2 inches from the tops of each pita round and discard. Open the pita to make a large pocket. Equally divide the shredded lettuce, tomato, and onion among the pita pockets. Equally divide the turkey among the pockets and top with equal amounts of the sour cream.

Patti's Pointers: Reduced-fat feta cheese is available in tubs in the refrigerated cheese case of most grocery stores. Athenos brand makes a good-tasting version that has ⅓ less fat than regular feta cheese.

Per Serving: 470 calories, 29 g protein, 43 g carbohydrate, 19 g fat, 10 g saturated fat, 110 mg cholesterol, 2 g dietary fiber, 760 mg sodium

Diet Exchanges: 3 lean meats, 2 fats, or 3 carbohydrate choices

Fabulous Fish
and Seafood

Crabmeat Quiche

This dish is a natural for Sunday brunch. Serve it with fresh fruit and the watercress salad on page 2 for a simple yet elegant meal.

Makes 8 servings

3 eggs
2 egg whites
1 cup fat-free half-and-half
1 tablespoon chopped fresh tarragon (optional)
½ teaspoon salt
⅛ teaspoon ground red pepper
½ cup shredded reduced-fat Swiss or mozzarella cheese
One 9-inch frozen pie shell
8 ounces jumbo lump crabmeat, picked over to remove shells
1 sprig fresh tarragon (optional)
Pinch of paprika (optional)

Preheat the oven to 325°F.

In a large bowl, whisk together the eggs, egg whites, half-and-half, tarragon (if using), salt, and ground red pepper. Whisk in the cheese.

Place the pie shell on a baking sheet. Arrange the crabmeat in the bottom of the pie shell. Pour the egg mixture on top.

Bake until set and a toothpick inserted in the center comes out clean, 40 to 45 minutes. Let cool (quiche should be warm, not hot) then (if using) garnish with the tarragon sprig and/or a dusting of paprika.

Option: If you have crab boil seasoning (such as Old Bay), use about 1¼ teaspoons of it in place of the salt and ground red pepper. It's the perfect flavoring for crab!

Patti's Pointers: If you can't find fresh jumbo lump crabmeat, look for premium handpicked pasteurized crabmeat in the seafood cold case. It comes in 8-ounce tubs and makes a good substitute.

Per Serving: 210 calories, 12 g protein, 16 g carbohydrate, 12 g fat, 1.5 g saturated fat, 115 mg cholesterol, 0 g dietary fiber, 560 mg sodium

Diet Exchanges: 2 meats, 1 starch, 2 fats, or 1½ carbohydrate choices

Seafood Marinara
with Angel-hair Pasta

8 ounces angel-hair pasta
2 tablespoons olive oil, divided
1 large onion, chopped
3 garlic cloves, minced
1 cup low-sodium chicken broth (about ½ of a 15-ounce can)
1 cup dry red wine
One 12-ounce can tomato paste
3 teaspoons dried Italian seasoning
½ teaspoon salt
6 large plum tomatoes, chopped (about 2 cups)
1 pound sea scallops, cut in half if large
1 pound mild white fish fillets, such as tilapia, or rockfish, cut into bite-size
  pieces
1 pound jumbo lump crabmeat, cleaned and picked over to remove shells
¼ cup chopped fresh basil
⅓ cup grated Parmesan cheese (optional)

Cook the pasta according to the package directions, leaving out any butter and salt.

Meanwhile, in a large saucepan over medium heat, warm 1 tablespoon of the olive oil. Add the onion and garlic and cook until tender, about 4 minutes. Stir in the broth, wine, tomato paste, Italian seasoning, and salt. Bring to a boil over high heat.

Reduce the heat to medium-low and add the tomatoes. Simmer, uncovered, for 10 to 15 minutes.

In a large skillet, warm the remaining 1 tablespoon of the olive oil. Add the scallops, fish, and crabmeat, and cook until the fish and scallops are just opaque, about 5 minutes. Transfer the seafood to the sauce and simmer for 5 minutes.

Serve over the pasta and sprinkle with the basil and Parmesan cheese (if using).

Patti's Pointers: If you can't find fresh jumbo lump crabmeat, look for premium handpicked pasteurized crabmeat in the seafood cold case. It comes in 8-ounce tubs and makes a good substitute. And, if you want to skip dirtying another pan, cook the seafood right in the sauce for about 5 minutes. The sauce will take on a stronger "fishier" flavor, but a lot of folks like it that way.

Per Serving: 360 calories, 37 g protein, 30 g carbohydrate, 9 g fat, 1.5 g saturated fat, 110 mg cholesterol, 3 g dietary fiber, 610 mg sodium

Diet Exchanges: 5 meats, 2 starches, 2 fats, or 2 carbohydrate choices

Pan-seared Flounder Fillets
with Corn and Tomato Sauce

I love fresh flounder fillets because they have such a mild, delicate, fresh-from-the-sea flavor. And, because they're so thin, they cook in a flash. Here's one of my favorite recipes for this fabulous fish. Try it; after one bite, I bet it will become one of your favorites, too.

Makes 4 servings

2 large ripe tomatoes, chopped (about 2 cups)
1 large shallot, chopped (about ¼ cup)
1 cup fresh or frozen sweet yellow corn
¼ cup dry white wine
2 teaspoons dried Italian seasoning
¾ teaspoon salt, divided
½ teaspoon freshly ground black pepper
Four 4-ounce flounder fillets
½ cup all-purpose flour
2 tablespoons extra-virgin olive oil
4 lemon wedges

In a shallow microwave-safe baking dish, combine the tomatoes, shallot, corn, wine, Italian seasoning, ¼ teaspoon of the salt, and ¼ teaspoon of the black pepper. Cover with a paper towel and microwave on medium just until steaming, about 2 minutes.

Wash fish in cold water and pat dry.

Sprinkle the fish with remaining ½ teaspoon salt and ¼ teaspoon black pepper. Dredge in the flour.

In a large heavy skillet, heat 1 tablespoon of the olive oil over medium-high heat until very hot. Place the fish in the skillet and cook until browned and just opaque on the underside, 2 to 3 minutes. Carefully flip with a spatula and cook the other side until just opaque, 2 to 3 minutes more. Remove the fish to a platter or plates.

Pour the tomato-corn mixture into the hot pan (it will spatter so stand back a bit). Let simmer for 1 to 2 minutes. Spoon the sauce over the fish and drizzle with the remaining 1 tablespoon olive oil. Serve with the lemon wedges for squeezing.

Option: You can use fresh, frozen, or canned corn in this recipe but you'll like the taste of fresh corn best. If using canned, you'll need one 8-ounce can, drained. If using fresh, you'll need the kernels from about 2 ears of corn.

Patti's Pointers: To cut kernels off the cob, cut off the stem end of each ear of corn to make a sturdy base. Hold an ear upright in a shallow bowl, standing the ear on its flat end. Using a sharp knife, cut straight down, slicing the kernels from the cob a few rows at a time. Don't cut too close to the cob. The kernels start to get tough closer to the cob.

Per Serving: 280 calories, 25 g protein, 25 g carbohydrate, 9 g fat, 1.5 g saturated fat, 55 mg cholesterol, 2 g dietary fiber, 550 mg sodium

Diet Exchanges: 3½ meats, 1½ starches, 2 fats, or 1½ carbohydrate choices

Party-Perfect Salmon Fillets in Parchment Paper

You know what's great about salmon? Other than the taste, I mean. It bakes like a dream with very little butter or oil. When I'm having a dinner party, I wrap it in parchment paper. It never fails to knock out my guests. Let them "unwrap" the salmon at the table. Martha Stewart won't have a thing on you.

Makes 6 servings

1 teaspoon olive oil
4 teaspoons fresh lemon juice
4 teaspoons chopped fresh dill
4 teaspoons chopped fresh tarragon
½ teaspoon salt
½ teaspoon ground black pepper
Six 4-ounce skinless salmon fillets
6 lemon wedges

Preheat the oven to 450°F.

Wash fish in cold water and pat dry.

In a small bowl, stir together the olive oil, lemon juice, dill, tarragon, salt, and pepper.

Tear off 6 large sheets of parchment paper, each at least twice as large as the fillets. Loosely fold a sheet in half and, starting at one of the folded corners, cut off the loose corners to make a heart shape. Repeat with remaining parchment.

Place each fillet on one half of each of the parchment hearts. Brush the fillets with the herbed mixture. Fold the parchment over the fish, bringing the opposite edges of the paper together. Make a series of tight double folds all the way around the edge of the paper. Overlap each fold to create a tight seal.

Put the packets on a large baking sheet and bake until the paper is lightly browned and puffed (if well sealed), about 15 minutes. The fish should be perfectly cooked at this point. If you're nervous about checking it for doneness, cut into your packet and slip a knife into the fish to see that it's just opaque throughout.

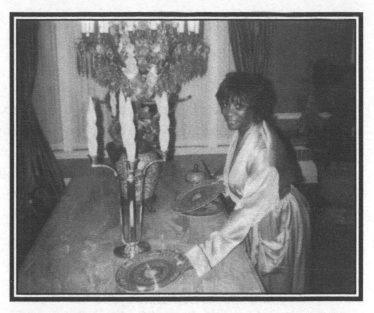

Setting the table before company arrives. I can't wait until they see what's for dinner!

To serve, place a packet on each plate and allow diners to slit open their packets individually. Serve with the lemon wedges for squeezing.

Patti's Pointers: If you don't have parchment paper, you can use foil. It's not as pretty, but works in a pinch. The French call this cooking method *en papillote,* which comes from the French word for butterfly, *papillon.* It refers to the traditional butterfly or heart shape that the parchment paper is cut into before sealing the food. If you don't want to bother with cutting heart shapes, you can just use rectangular sheets of parchment or foil, bring the long edges together, fold them down tightly over the fish, then tuck the short edges underneath. It's not nearly as impressive, but works fine. And as long as you have the oven on, roast some asparagus (see recipe on page 154) for a side dish that's the perfect complement to this wonderful fish.

Per Serving: 170 calories, 23 g protein, 2 g carbohydrate, 8 g fat, 1 g saturated fat, 60 mg cholesterol, 0 g dietary fiber, 240 mg sodium

Diet Exchanges: 3 meats, 1½ fats, or 0 carbohydrate choices

Herbed Grilled Tuna

Tuna is my favorite fish for grilling. Tuna and charcoal go together like hard-shell crabs and beer. And it freezes like a dream so, unlike a lot of other fish, you can buy tuna frozen and not worry about losing any of the flavor. While you can broil it (place it about 4 inches from the heat source), it's so fly-you-to-the-moon good on the grill that my advice is to wait until you're cooking out to try this recipe. The wait will be worth it; everybody knows that, in the summer, the best cooking is done in a kitchen with a ceiling made of sky.

Makes 4 servings

3 tablespoons fresh lemon juice
1 tablespoon chopped fresh parsley
1 tablespoon chopped fresh oregano
1 tablespoon chopped fresh chives
1 teaspoon coarse kosher salt
1 tablespoon Dijon mustard
1 large garlic clove, minced
¼ teaspoon red pepper flakes
Four 6-ounce tuna steaks, each about 1 inch thick

Preheat the grill to hot.

In a small bowl, stir together the lemon juice, parsley, oregano, chives, salt, mustard, garlic, and red pepper flakes. Brush onto the tuna.

Grill the steaks until lightly browned on the underside, 2 to 4 minutes. Turn with tongs and grill until browned on the other side, 2 to 4 minutes, more for medium-rare. The steaks should still be pink in the center. To check, separate the center of the flesh with tongs or make a small slit with a paring knife.

Patti's Pointers: As long as you've got the grill going, throw on some rough-cut vegetables like red bell peppers, zucchini, and onions tossed with olive oil, salt, and pepper. They make a wonderful accompaniment to the tuna.

Per Serving: 250 calories, 40 g protein, 2 g carbohydrate, 9 g fat, 2 g saturated fat, 65 mg cholesterol, 0 g dietary fiber, 740 mg sodium

Diet Exchanges: 5 meats, 1 fat, or 0 carbohydrate choices

Slammin' Seafood Bouillabaisse

Serve this classic fisherman's soup when company's coming. I promise: they will be impressed!

Makes 8 servings

1 tablespoon olive oil
1½ cups chopped red onion
4 garlic cloves, minced
1 teaspoon ground cumin
½ teaspoon ground red pepper (or more if, like me, you like it hot, hot, hot!)
2 cups reduced-sodium chicken broth or vegetable broth
2 cups dry white wine
1 red tomato, chopped
1 yellow tomato, chopped (total tomatoes should equal 2 cups)
½ teaspoon salt
1 teaspoon dried thyme
2 bay leaves
1 large pinch saffron threads, crushed
1 pound medium fresh shrimp, peeled and deveined (leave the tail on; it's cute)
1 pound sea scallops, cut in half if they are large
1 pound cod or grouper fillet cut into bite-size pieces
1 pound catfish fillets, cut into bite-size pieces
12 snow crab cocktail claws

In a large stew pot, heat the olive oil over medium heat. Add the onion and garlic and cook until tender, about 4 minutes.

Stir in the cumin and red pepper and cook 1 minute.

Stir in the broth, wine, red tomato, yellow tomato, salt, thyme, bay leaves, and saffron. Simmer, uncovered, for about 15 minutes.

Wash the seafood in cold water and pat dry. Add it to the broth mixture and bring to a boil over high heat. Reduce the heat to low, cover, and simmer until the seafood is just opaque, 10 to 15 minutes.

Option: Serve this dish over cooked rice. You'll need about 4 cups cooked, which is about 2 cups dry.

Patti's Pointers: Be sure to use snow crab cocktail claws. Not only are they much easier to eat than Alaskan king crab legs, they also help cut down on the sodium. (Just two Alaskan king crab legs can have more than 2,000 mg of sodium!)

Per Serving: 310 calories, 45 g protein, 6 g carbohydrate, 6 g fat, 1.5 g saturated fat, 200 mg cholesterol, less than 1 g dietary fiber, 540 mg sodium

Diet Exchanges: 6 meats, 1 fat, or ½ carbohydrate choice

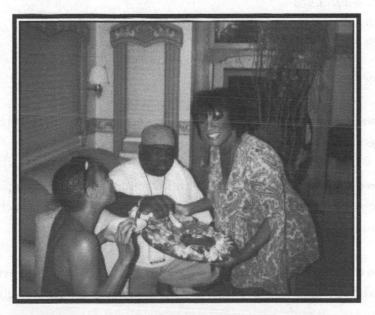

Serving shrimp before dinner to friends who insisted they couldn't wait for the main event.

Champagne Sautéed Sea Scallops

There's just one rule to follow to ensure that this dish turns out perfectly every time: don't overcook the scallops! We're going for yummy, not yucky and—trust me—yucky (i.e., rubbery as a tire) is just what you get when you overcook scallops. And if you're worried about the champagne in the recipe, don't. Most of the alcohol evaporates at high temperatures. For instance, a half cup of champagne or wine added to a hot pan will boil off in about one minute, leaving you with all the flavor without all the calories and fat. Now if I could just figure out how to do that with macaroni and cheese!

Makes 4 servings

1 tablespoon reduced-calorie margarine
3 small garlic cloves, minced
½ cup champagne or dry white wine
1½ pounds sea scallops
½ teaspoon salt
½ teaspoon freshly ground black pepper
1 tablespoon chopped fresh basil or dill
4 lemon wedges

Melt the margarine in a large skillet over medium heat. Add the garlic and cook until just golden, about 2 minutes.

Pour in the champagne and cook until warm, 1 minute. Add the scallops and cook until just opaque throughout, about 3 minutes per side, sprinkling each side with the salt and black pepper during cooking.

Transfer to a platter or plates and spoon some of the cooking liquid over the top. Sprinkle with the basil or dill and serve with the lemon wedges for squeezing.

Option: These taste fabulous over angel-hair pasta (you'll need 2 cups cooked, which is about 4 ounces dry). To moisten and flavor the pasta, toss it with the cooking liquid from the scallops.

Patti's Pointers: For the best flavor, look for "dry" or "unsoaked" sea scallops. Because scallop boats stay out at sea for weeks at a time, to preserve them, many fishermen soak sea scallops in a solution of sodium tripolyphosphate (don't even think about asking me to pronounce it). It makes the scallops last longer but increases the weight (and the price) and dilutes the flavor. Next time you're at the fish market, ask if your scallops are dry or soaked. Or take a close look at them. Soaked scallops are bright and shiny, and cling together in clumps. Dry scallops are pale ivory or pale coral in color and usually remain separate.

Per Serving: 200 calories, 29 g protein, 6 g carbohydrate, 4 g fat, 1 g saturated fat, 55 mg cholesterol, 0 g dietary fiber, 600 mg sodium

Diet Exchanges: 4 meats, ½ starch, 1 fat, or ½ carbohydrate choice

Sublime Seafood Grill

You know how, back in the sixties, whenever people talked about the Beatles, Paul was known as the cute one? Well, back in my old neighborhood, whenever people talked about the Holte girls, my sister Barbara was known as the sweet one. (Vivian was the beautiful one, Jackie was the fiery one, and I was the shy one who could sing.) And Barbara *was* sweet. Just as sweet as sugar. If you hit her, Barbara would ask you if you had hurt your hand. That's just the kind of person she was. She didn't have a mean bone in her body.

And you know what else I loved about Barbara? The way she looked at life. Like every day—every hour—was an incredible gift. Her outlook was so amazing, so affirmative, so cool. Not like she didn't know upsetting things were happening, more like she didn't trip about it. More than anyone I have ever known, Barbara focused on the good in everything and everybody.

I was performing on Broadway when the colon cancer that killed Barbara started to make her sicker than sick. Can't-get-out-the-bed sick. Hold-my-hand-until-I-fall-asleep sick. But since I couldn't hold Barbara's hand, at least not physically, I held it via telephone. Until she was hospitalized, I sang her a song she loved every single day.

As much as Barbara loved that song, she loved herself some seafood. I mean she had a thing for it. She was tiny as she could be—I'm talking size-6 tiny. But she could put away some seafood. Whenever Chubby cooked it, Barbara was the first one at the table. One minute her plate would be full and the next it would be clean enough to satisfy the Board of Health. You know what else Barbara loved? Our outdoor barbecues. She looked forward to them the way a kid looks forward to Christmas. In her honor, this recipe combines what she loved about both.

Makes 6 servings

2 tablespoons reduced-calorie margarine, melted
1½ teaspoons salt-free lemon-pepper seasoning
½ teaspoon salt
¼ teaspoon red pepper flakes
1 pound skinless mahimahi fillets, cut into
*   1½-inch pieces*
1 pound medium fresh shrimp, peeled and
*   deveined, tails left on*
1 pound tilapia fillets, cut into 1½-inch
*   pieces*
2 tablespoons chopped fresh parsley
6 lemon wedges

Preheat the grill to medium-high and coat a grill basket with fat-free cooking spray.

In a large bowl, combine the margarine, lemon-pepper seasoning, salt, and red pepper flakes. Add the seafood to the bowl and toss to coat.

My beloved sister Barbara on her wedding day. She was as beautiful a person as she was a bride.

Place the seafood in a single layer in the prepared grill basket. Put the basket on the grill grate and grill, turning once, until the seafood is just opaque, 10 to 15 minutes. (Don't overcook! That's the second-biggest secret to great-tasting fish.) Sprinkle with the parsley and serve with the lemon wedges for squeezing.

Patti's Pointers: If you don't have a grill basket, not to worry. Just coat a couple of disposable aluminum pans with fat-free cooking spray and use them instead. No aluminum pans handy either? Then wrap the fish in heavy-duty aluminum foil sprayed with fat-free cooking spray and throw it on the grill. To get that great grilled flavor, be sure to poke several holes in the foil with a fork. (I think charcoal gives the best grilled flavor here, but this recipe can be done on a gas grill. To boost the flavor, soak hickory wood chips in water for 30 minutes, then toss them on the central plate of your gas grill and close the cover during cooking.)

Per Serving: 270 calories, 44 g protein, 1 g carbohydrate, 9 g fat, 1.5 g saturated fat, 210 mg cholesterol, 0 g dietary fiber, 480 mg sodium

Diet Exchanges: 6 meats, 2 fats, or 0 carbohydrate choices

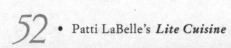

Succulent Steamed Sea Bass
with Broccoli, Mushrooms, and Summer Squash

The steam gives the fish a moist and tender texture and cooks the vegetables perfectly—not too crispy, not too soggy. And because you cook all the ingredients in aluminum foil, cleanup is super easy and super fast. Twenty minutes after you pop this concoction in the oven, unwrap the foil and announce, "Dinner's ready."

Makes 6 servings

Six 4-ounce sea bass fillets
¾ teaspoon salt
¼ teaspoon ground white or black pepper
1 tablespoon chopped fresh basil or parsley
½ cup thinly sliced broccoli florets
½ cup sliced fresh mushrooms
½ thinly sliced yellow squash
1 tablespoon reduced-calorie margarine
6 lemon wedges

Preheat the oven to 450°F. Tear off a sheet of heavy-duty aluminum foil that is large enough to hold all ingredients comfortably (about 2 feet long). Coat the foil with fat-free cooking spray.

Put the fish in the center of the foil and sprinkle with half of the salt, pepper, and basil or parsley. Top with the broccoli, mushrooms, and squash. Sprinkle with the remaining salt, pepper, and basil or parsley. Dot with pieces of the margarine.

Bring together the long sides of the foil and fold down tightly over the fish. Fold up the short sides of the foil.

Put the packet on a baking sheet and bake until the fish is just opaque, 18 to 20 minutes (it's okay to open the packet to check that the fish is opaque all the way through).

Patti's Pointers: Don't feel you *have* to use broccoli, mushrooms, and squash in this recipe. Whatever is fresh and in season—tomatoes, zucchini, corn—will work just fine, probably better. That goes double for the fish; you can use any fish with dense, tender flesh and a delicate flavor, like sea trout or cod.

Per Serving: 130 calories, 19 g protein, 3 g carbohydrate, 4 g fat, 1 g saturated fat, 40 mg cholesterol, 1 g dietary fiber, 390 mg sodium

Diet Exchanges: 2½ meats, 1 fat, or 0 carbohydrate choices

Magnificent Monkfish
with Caramelized Onions and Olives

If you ever saw a monkfish, you'd probably never eat one. It's probably the ugliest fish in the sea, I kid you not! A monkfish has a humongous head and an even bigger mouth. It's so big and ugly that fishermen usually keep the tail end of the monkfish and throw away the head and body. Ugly as it is, however, monkfish is as heavenly tasting as it is hideous-looking. Serve this recipe with the squash and sweet onions on page 157 and I guarantee you won't have to fish for compliments.

Makes 4 servings

4 teaspoons margarine, divided
2 Vidalia or other sweet onions, thinly sliced
¼ teaspoon salt
½ teaspoon freshly ground black pepper
¼ cup pitted Kalamata olives
¼ teaspoon ground red pepper
1 pound monkfish fillets, membrane removed (see Patti's Pointers below)
2 tablespoons chopped fresh parsley
4 lemon wedges

Coat a very large skillet with fat-free cooking spray and heat over medium-high heat. Melt 3 teaspoons of the margarine in the skillet and stir in the onions, separating them into rings.

Cook and stir until softened, 2 to 3 minutes. Sprinkle with the salt and ¼ teaspoon of the pepper. Reduce the heat to medium-low, cover, and cook, stirring occasionally, until the onions are deep brown, about 15 minutes. Stir in the olives. Remove the mixture to a plate and cover with foil to keep warm.

In a small bowl, combine the red pepper and remaining ¼ teaspoon black pepper. Cut the fish crosswise into 1-inch-thick medallions. Rub the spice mixture evenly into both sides of the medallions.

Melt the remaining 1 teaspoon margarine over medium heat in the same skillet used to cook the onions. When hot, add the medallions and cook until opaque throughout, about 3 minutes per side.

Remove to a platter or plates and top with the onion mixture. Sprinkle with the parsley and serve with the lemon wedges for squeezing.

Patti's Pointers: Ask your fishmonger to thoroughly trim the monkfish fillets. That means cutting away the pinkish-gray inner membrane. If you happen to see any grayish membrane covering your fillets, it's easy to cut it away yourself. Just slip a knife underneath it where it attaches to the fillet and cut it off with horizontal sawing motions. You may see a narrow, dark red fatty strip that runs the length of the fillet (which is actually the tail of the fish). It's okay to leave that on. But if it bothers you, feel free to trim off that dark red strip, too.

Per Serving: 180 calories, 17 g protein, 6 g carbohydrate, 9 g fat, 1.5 g saturated fat, 30 mg cholesterol, 1 g dietary fiber, 450 mg sodium

Diet Exchanges: 2 meats, 2 fats, ½ starch, or ½ carbohydrate choice

Scrumptious and Simple Scrod in "Butter" and Basil Sauce

Believe it or not, scrod isn't actually a type of fish like whiting and sea bass and catfish. I don't know who came up with the name or why, since fish markets use the term "scrod" to describe *all kinds* of fish—from cod to cusk, haddock to pollock. My professional fisherman friends tell me that, more often than not, fish labeled "scrod" is actually some type of mild white fillet. So, when purchasing fish labeled "scrod," don't shell out a whole bunch of money thinking you're getting some exotic and unique species from the sea. Just keep in mind what matters most: *freshness!*

Makes 4 servings

Four 4-ounce scrod fillets
2 tablespoons margarine
1 garlic clove, minced
¼ teaspoon salt
¼ teaspoon imitation butter-flavor salt, such as Molly McButter
⅛ teaspoon red pepper flakes
2 tablespoons chopped fresh basil
4 lemon wedges

Preheat the oven to 450°F. and coat a baking sheet with fat-free cooking spray.

Wash the fish in cold water and pat dry.

Place the margarine in a medium bowl and melt in the microwave, about 15 seconds. Stir in the garlic, salt, imitation butter-flavor salt, red pepper flakes, and basil.

Brush the butter mixture all over the fish. Place on the prepared baking sheet and bake until the fish is just opaque throughout, 5 to 7 minutes. Serve with the lemon wedges for squeezing.

Per Serving: 190 calories, 22 g protein, 2 g carbohydrate, 10 g fat, 2 g saturated fat, 75 mg cholesterol, 0 g dietary fiber, 450 mg sodium

Diet Exchanges: 3 meats, 2 fats, or 0 carbohydrate choices

Savory Shrimp Scampi

Fair warning: This dish will have folks showing up at your doorstep—unannounced, uninvited, unembarrassed—if they find out you're making it. When you serve it, don't tell anyone that it's a lite version of this classic and delicious Southern European dish. Instead, tell everybody it was passed down to you from your great-great grandmother on your daddy's side. And while you'd love to share the recipe, before it was passed down to *you,* you had to take an oath of secrecy to keep it in the family. That little story will make it taste even better!

Makes 4 servings

2 tablespoons reduced-calorie margarine
1 tablespoon olive oil
4 garlic cloves, minced
1 pound fresh shrimp, peeled and deveined
½ cup dry white wine
3 tablespoons fresh lemon juice
¼ teaspoon salt
¼ teaspoon salt-free lemon-pepper seasoning
¼ teaspoon white pepper
¼ teaspoon red pepper flakes
3 tablespoons chopped fresh parsley

In a large skillet over medium heat, melt the margarine and olive oil. Add the garlic and cook, stirring frequently, for 1 minute.

Add the shrimp and cook until they just begin to turn pink, 1 to 2 minutes. Add the wine, lemon juice, salt, lemon-pepper seasoning, white pepper, and red pepper flakes. Reduce the heat to medium-low and cook until the wine reduces by almost half. Sprinkle with the parsley and serve piping hot.

Option: This tastes great over cooked angel-hair pasta or white rice. You'll need about 2 cups of either one.

Per Serving: 170 calories, 18 g protein, 2 g carbohydrate, 8 g fat, 1.5 g saturated fat, 160 mg cholesterol, 0 g dietary fiber, 400 mg sodium

Diet Exchanges: 2½ meats, 1½ fats, or 0 carbohydrate choices

No-Fuss Blackened Fish Fillets

I like to make this dish using grouper, but it works just as well with any mild white fish, like tilapia or ocean perch. I've found it cooks best in a big old cast-iron skillet—the kind Grandmother Ellen used to fry her famous fried chicken in.

Makes 4 servings

1 pound fish fillets, such as grouper, tilapia, or ocean perch
2 tablespoons blackening seasoning
1 teaspoon dried thyme
1 teaspoon paprika
½ teaspoon freshly ground black pepper
¼ teaspoon ground red pepper
1 tablespoon canola oil
4 lemon wedges

Wash the fish in cold water and pat dry.

Sprinkle the fish with the blackening seasoning, thyme, paprika, black pepper, and ground red pepper, patting it in on both sides.

Coat a large cast-iron skillet or other heavy-bottomed skillet with fat-free cooking spray. Add the oil and heat over medium-high heat until smoking hot. Put the fish in the pan and cook, turning once, until just opaque throughout, about 2 minutes per side.

Serve with the lemon wedges for squeezing.

Patti's Pointers: This dish creates a bit of smoke, so turn on your overhead fan or open the window!

Per Serving: 140 calories, 22 g protein, 1 g carbohydrate, 4.5 g fat, 0.5 g saturated fat, 40 mg cholesterol, 0 g dietary fiber, 640 mg sodium

Diet Exchanges: 3 meats, 1 fat, or 0 carbohydrate choices

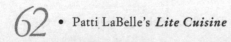

Crunchy Cajun Catfish Nuggets

Let me say this from the start: This Cajun classic is for folks who like their food hot and spicy—the more of each the better. If, like me, you happen to be a life-long member of this club, I've got one word for you: rejoice! Recent studies have shown that hot peppers may have serious health benefits—and rev up your metabolism to boot. Who knew? All I can say is, "Bring on the hot pepper sauce, sugar."

Makes 6 servings

¾ cup plain dry bread crumbs
½ teaspoon Cajun or Creole seasoning
1 teaspoon chili powder
¼ teaspoon ground red pepper
Six 4-ounce catfish fillets, cut into bite-size pieces
Hot pepper sauce, such as Tabasco
6 lemon wedges

Preheat the oven to 425°F.

Line a cookie sheet with foil and coat with fat-free cooking spray.

In a large shallow bowl, mix together the bread crumbs, Cajun or Creole seasoning, chili powder, and ground red pepper.

Coat the catfish nuggets with cooking spray. Dip the nuggets in bread-crumb mixture, rolling to coat completely.

Preheat the cookie sheet in the oven until smoking hot, 2 to 3 minutes. (A hot cookie sheet helps make the nuggets crunchier, giving them that real "Southern fried" taste.) Place the nuggets on the hot cookie sheet, coat the tops with fat-free cooking spray, and bake until just opaque throughout, about 12 minutes.

Serve drizzled with hot pepper sauce and with the lemon wedges for squeezing.

Option: These taste fabulous with reduced-fat blue cheese or ranch dressing.

Per Serving: 170 calories, 20 g protein, 11 g carbohydrate, 4 g fat, 1 g saturated fat, 65 mg cholesterol, less than 1 g dietary fiber, 250 mg sodium

Diet Exchanges: 3 meats, 1 starch, 1 fat, or 1 carbohydrate choice

Oh-So-Good Orange Roughy
with Roasted Tomato and Olive Relish

Makes 4 servings

4 large plum tomatoes, halved lengthwise
Four 4-ounce orange roughy fillets
¼ teaspoon salt
¼ teaspoon freshly ground black pepper
1 tablespoon olive oil
¼ cup sliced pimiento-stuffed green olives, drained
One 4-ounce can chopped green chilis, drained
1 tablespoon chopped fresh oregano or 1 teaspoon dried
4 lemon wedges

Position an oven rack in the top third of the oven and preheat the oven to 425°F. Coat a 13 × 9-inch baking dish with fat-free olive oil–flavored cooking spray.

Place the tomatoes cut side up in the prepared baking dish and roast in the top third of the oven until lightly browned on top, 10 to 15 minutes. Remove to a cutting board, chop, and transfer to a bowl with all the juices.

Meanwhile, wash the fish in cold water and pat dry. Coat with fat-free olive oil–flavored cooking spray on both sides. Sprinkle with ⅛ teaspoon of the salt and ⅛ teaspoon of the pepper. Place in the baking dish and cook until just opaque throughout, 8 to 10 minutes.

Add the olive oil, olives, and green chilis to the bowl with the tomatoes. Stir in the oregano, remaining ⅛ teaspoon salt, and remaining ⅛ teaspoon pepper.

Transfer the fish to plates if desired. Spoon the tomato relish evenly over the fillets. Serve with the lemon wedges for squeezing.

Per Serving: 150 calories, 18 g protein, 10 g carbohydrate, 5 g fat, 0.5 g saturated fat, 25 mg cholesterol, 2 g dietary fiber, 330 mg sodium

Diet Exchanges: 2½ meats, 1 fat, ½ starch, or ½ carbohydrate choice

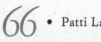

Crab Imperial

This is another great "company's coming" dish that is guaranteed to impress your guests. Serve it for a special Sunday supper and sit back and bask in the compliments.

Makes 8 servings

2 teaspoons regular margarine
½ cup finely chopped celery
½ cup finely chopped red bell pepper
½ cup finely chopped yellow bell pepper
3 tablespoons chopped fresh tarragon
1 teaspoon Dijon mustard
¼ teaspoon freshly ground black pepper
¼ teaspoon red pepper flakes
2 eggs
⅓ cup reduced-fat mayonnaise, such as Hellmann's Just 2 Good!
1½ teaspoon crab boil seasoning, such as Old Bay
1½ pounds fresh jumbo lump crabmeat, picked over to remove shells

Preheat the oven to 375°F.

Melt the margarine in a large skillet over medium heat. Add the celery, red pepper, and yellow pepper. Cook, stirring occasionally, until tender, about 4 minutes.

Remove from the heat and stir in the tarragon, Dijon mustard, black pepper, and red pepper flakes.

In a medium bowl, whisk together the eggs and mayonnaise until smooth. Whisk in 1 teaspoon of the crab boil seasoning. Set aside ⅓ cup of the egg mixture.

Using your hands or a rubber spatula, gently fold the crabmeat into the remaining egg mixture, being careful not to break up the lumps of crab. Divide the mixture equally among 8 ramekins or custard cups sprayed with fat-free cooking spray. Spread 2 teaspoons of the reserved egg mixture over the top of each ramekin or cup. Sprinkle with the remaining ½ teaspoon crab boil seasoning evenly distributed over each ramekin or cup. Place on a baking sheet and bake until just slightly crisp on top, about 20 minutes.

Option: For an extra-crisp topping, sprinkle each serving with 2 teaspoons dry bread crumbs (⅓ cup total) before baking.

Patti's Pointers: Restaurants often serve this dish in emptied upside-down crab shells instead of ramekins. Ask your fishmonger if he has leftover crab shells. They make a drop-dead cute presentation! If you can't find these and don't have ramekins, you can also bake this in a single 10-inch pie plate, then divide the servings at the table.

Per Serving: 150 calories, 19 g protein, 3 g carbohydrate, 6 g fat, 1 g saturated fat, 140 mg cholesterol, 0 g dietary fiber, 560 mg sodium

Diet Exchanges: 2½ meats, 1 fat, 1 vegetable, or 0 carbohydrate choices

Rockin' Rockfish

True fish connoisseurs say that rockfish, also called striped bass, is the best eating fish on the planet. That's because of the flesh; it's the perfect combination of moist, sweet, lean, and firm. That's why I've kept this recipe simple. The rockfish is so full of flavor it needs no dressing up. If you're in the mood for a barbecue, it's also one of the few fish that is firm enough to cook on the grill without falling apart. Either way you cook it, it will be off the hook.

Makes 4 servings

Four 5-ounce rockfish (striped bass) fillets, each about ¾ inch thick
1 teaspoon dried thyme
1 teaspoon ground cumin
1 teaspoon paprika
½ teaspoon garlic powder
⅓ teaspoon salt
¾ teaspoon freshly ground black pepper
4 lemon wedges

Preheat the oven to 450°F. Coat a roasting pan with fat-free cooking spray.

Wash the fish in cold water and pat dry. Lay the fish in the prepared pan, skin side down.

In a small bowl, mix together the thyme, cumin, paprika, garlic powder, salt, and black pepper. Sprinkle over the fish and pat into the flesh with your hands. Coat the tops with fat-free cooking spray.

Roast until just opaque throughout, 8 to 10 minutes. Using a spatula, lift from the roasting pan onto a platter or plates. Serve with the lemon wedges for squeezing.

Patti's Pointers: If you like fish with crisp skin, preheat the roasting pan in the oven until hot, 2 to 3 minutes. Season the fish on a piece of waxed paper or foil, then place skin side down in the hot pan. Continue roasting as directed.

Per Serving: 180 calories, 34 g protein, 2 g carbohydrate, 3 g fat, 0.5 g saturated fat, 60 mg cholesterol, 0 g dietary fiber, 300 mg sodium

Diet Exchanges: 5 meats, ½ fat, or 0 carbohydrate choices

The Perfect Porgy

I would love to claim credit for this divine recipe but I can't. It was given to me by professional fishermen on the island of Eleuthera. That's where I go when my life gets too crazy and I need to cool out. It's such a calm and peaceful place. When I'm on the island, I do absolutely nothing but sleep (like a baby), look at the ocean (for hours at a time), and cook (just about every day). Still, it took me more than a year to try this recipe. That's because when I saw all the salt that was in it, I thought I would end up with a soggy, salty, *seriously awful* mess. Boy, was I ever wrong. The salt in this recipe acts as insulation; you actually tap off and discard the entire salt crust before serving. But when the fish is *cooking,* the salt works a little culinary magic, sealing in the juices of the fish and creating the moistest flesh I have ever tasted. So, to my fisherman friends in Eleuthera, thanks a million for turning me on to the easiest, most foolproof recipe I know for cooking whole fish. And one of the most delicious to boot!

Makes 4 servings

Two 1½-pound whole porgies, cleaned, scaled, and dressed
2 teaspoons reduced-calorie margarine, melted
¼ teaspoon freshly ground black pepper
6 sprigs fresh oregano
4 lemon slices
4 egg whites
2 cups coarse kosher salt
4 teaspoons extra-virgin olive oil
4 lemon wedges

Preheat the oven to 450°F. Choose a 13 × 9-inch baking dish or other 3-quart baking dish that can double as a serving platter. Line the baking dish with foil.

Rinse the fish inside and out in cold water and pat dry. Brush the margarine inside the cavity of the fish. Sprinkle the cavity evenly with the pepper. Stuff the oregano sprigs and lemon slices inside.

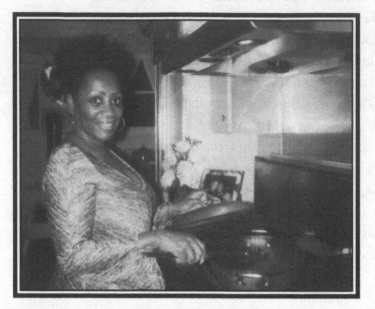

Getting set up to prepare the Perfect Porgy.

In a large bowl, whisk the egg whites until soft peaks form when the whisk is lifted. Fold in the salt.

Spread one-third of the salt mixture in the bottom of the prepared pan. Place the fish on the salt and cover the top of the fish with the remaining salt mixture.

Bake for 30 minutes. Tap off and discard the salt crust from the fish (it will break off easily). Drizzle the fish with the olive oil and serve in its baking dish with the lemon wedges for squeezing. To make individual portions, cut the fish into quarters and remove to plates. To remove the skin, peel it off with a fork.

Patti's Pointers: If porgies aren't fresh at your market (or that's not what you've caught), you can also use whole red snapper or sea bass. You'll need about 3 pounds total. Be sure to thoroughly clean and scale the fish so that it can be baked whole. To get this kind of service from your fishmonger, call ahead and tell him exactly what you need. To clean a whole fish yourself, begin by gutting it. Using a sharp knife, slit the belly from the gills to the anal fin. Pull out and discard the organs. Scrape any dark blood from the backbone area. Rinse the cavity with cold running water.

Next, remove the scales and gills. Hold the fish underwater by the tail. Scrape the scales forward from tail to head using a fish scaler or the dull back edge of a fillet knife. Open the gill flaps on each side of the fish to expose the dark red crescent-shaped gills. Using kitchen shears or scissors, cut the cartilage at each end of the gills, then pull out and discard the gills.

Now you can "dress" the fish, which means removing the fins and head. If you prefer the look of a whole cooked fish with the head, leave the head on. Otherwise, use a large chef's knife to cut off the head on an angle behind the gill opening and pectoral fin. Cut off all the fins with the knife or kitchen shears. Now your fish is ready for baking.

Per Serving: 290 calories, 46 g protein, 3 g carbohydrate, 9 g fat, 1.5 g saturated fat, 110 mg cholesterol, less than 1 g dietary fiber, 400 mg sodium

Diet Exchanges: 6½ meats, 2 fats, or 0 carbohydrate choices

Hellacious Halibut
with Lemon and Cilantro

While I love the taste of halibut, when cooked in the oven it has a tendency to dry out. So to make sure these steaks come out just the way they should—moist and magnificent—I spray them with fat-free cooking spray before pouring the margarine on top. Give it a try—you're gonna love the result.

Makes 4 servings

Four 6-ounce halibut steaks
1 tablespoon reduced-calorie margarine, melted
2 tablespoons fresh lemon juice
¾ teaspoon salt-free lemon-pepper seasoning
½ teaspoon coarse kosher salt
1 tablespoon chopped fresh cilantro or 1 teaspoon dried
4 lemon wedges

Preheat the oven to 450°F. and coat a shallow 2-quart baking dish with fat-free cooking spray.

Wash the fish in cold water and pat dry. Coat the fish all over with fat-free cooking spray. Put into the prepared baking dish and pour the margarine evenly over the top. Sprinkle with the lemon juice, lemon-pepper seasoning, and salt.

Bake until the fish is just opaque, 20 to 25 minutes. Sprinkle with the cilantro before serving with the lemon wedges for squeezing.

Patti's Pointers: Don't be thrown off if the halibut at your store is labeled "boneless fillets." As long as they're at least 1 inch thick, they can be used just like a halibut steak.

Per Serving: 220 calories, 36 g protein, 2 g carbohydrate, 7 g fat, 1.5 g saturated fat, 55 mg cholesterol, 0 g dietary fiber, 420 mg sodium

Diet Exchanges: 5 meats, 1 fat, or 0 carbohydrate choices

Melt-in-Your-Mouth
Meat Dishes

Veal Parmigiana

Unlike beef, you don't have to be too worried about picking a specific cut of veal, since most cuts are considered lean. That's because veal comes from young animals and doesn't have the fat you find in other good cuts of meat. So choose whatever cut you're feeling, as the teenagers would say. Leg, shoulder, sirloin—they will all work. When I created this recipe, I was feeling cutlets. But whatever you select, this dish will be lean *and* luscious.

Makes 4 servings

1 pound veal cutlets
½ cup egg substitute, such as Egg Beaters
½ cup dry Italian-seasoned bread crumbs
One 8-ounce can reduced-sodium tomato sauce
2 tablespoons chopped fresh basil or 1 teaspoon dried
½ cup shredded reduced-fat mozzarella cheese

Preheat the oven to 450°F.

Put a veal cutlet between two sheets of waxed paper on a work surface. Using a rolling pin or heavy pan, gently pound the cutlet from the center outward until it is between ⅛ inch and ¼ inch thick. Repeat with the remaining cutlets.

Pour the egg substitute into a shallow bowl.

Put the bread crumbs in another shallow bowl.

Dip the cutlets in the egg substitute, then in bread crumbs, coating completely.

Coat a large skillet with fat-free cooking spray and heat over medium-high heat. Add the cutlets (in batches if necessary) and cook until browned, about 2 minutes per side.

Transfer the cutlets to a shallow baking dish. Pour the tomato sauce evenly over the top. Sprinkle with the basil and cheese.

Bake until the cutlets are no longer pink in the center and the cheese is melted, about 12 to 15 minutes.

Option: Of course, pasta makes a natural accompaniment here. You'll need about 2 cups uncooked total.

Patti's Pointers: When shopping for veal, look for meat that's quite pale, with creamy white fat. A pale color means that the veal has been milk-fed rather than grass-fed or grain-fed. And that means more tender meat for you. If you see a reddish tinge to the meat, pass it up. A reddish tinge means that the cut came from an older calf that may have been grain-fed; and most likely the meat is less tender in texture and less delicate in flavor.

Per Serving: 330 calories, 31 g protein, 16 g carbohydrate, 15 g fat, 6 g saturated fat, 85 mg cholesterol, 2 g dietary fiber, 590 mg sodium

Diet Exchanges: 4 medium-fat meats, 1 starch, or 1 carbohydrate choice

Verrrry Good Veal Chops
with Mushroom Gravy

Makes 4 servings

Four 4-ounce veal loin chops
½ teaspoon salt
½ teaspoon ground black pepper
2 onions, thinly sliced and separated into rings
2 garlic cloves, minced
½ cup fat-free chicken broth
1½ cups sliced fresh mushrooms
½ cup reduced-fat sour cream
1 tablespoon chopped fresh thyme or ½ teaspoon dried

Sprinkle the veal chops with ¼ teaspoon of the salt and ¼ teaspoon of the pepper.

Coat a large skillet with fat-free cooking spray and heat over medium-high heat until smoking hot. Add the chops and cook until browned all over, 1 to 2 minutes per side. Remove to a plate.

Reduce the heat to medium and add the onions to the skillet. Cook until very soft, about 5 minutes. Add the garlic and cook 2 minutes longer.

Reduce the heat to medium-low and return the chops to the skillet. Pour the broth over the top, cover, and simmer until the veal is slightly pink in the center and registers 140°F on an instant-read thermometer, 8 to 10 minutes.

Remove the veal and onions to a platter or plates, creating a bed of onions and putting the veal on top. Cover with foil to keep warm.

Add the mushrooms to the skillet and cook over low heat until tender, about 5 minutes. Stir in the sour cream, thyme, remaining ¼ teaspoon salt and remaining ¼ teaspoon pepper. Cook until heated through, about 2 minutes. Pour the mushroom gravy over the veal and onions before serving.

Patti's Pointers: Button mushrooms work fine in this recipe, but go wild if you want. Fresh wild mushrooms like shiitakes, creminis, or morels take this dish to a whole new level.

Per Serving: 190 calories, 18 g protein, 8 g carbohydrates, 9 g fat, 5 g saturated fat, 65 mg cholesterol, 1 g dietary fiber, 400 mg sodium

Diet Exchanges: 2 medium-fat meats, 1 vegetable, or ½ carbohydrate choice

Seven-Layer Beef Skillet

If you've got kids in the house, let them help you make this dish. They love fixing it almost as much as they love eating it. And they *love* eating it—it's like home-made Hamburger Helper and not much harder to make. Take it from someone who, as a kid, practically lived in her mother's kitchen: just hanging out with you and cooking together will make your kid feel good. When Whoopi Goldberg's granddaughter was only nine, Whoopi said her granddaughter loved it when the two of them concocted dishes together. And we're not talking Jell-O-and-whipped-cream-peanut-butter-and-bananas kinds of concoctions either. Oh, no. At nine, little girlfriend was into *sautéing*. I have just two things to say: "You go, girl!" And, Whoopi, the next time your granddaughter is cooking, can I come over for dinner?

Makes 8 servings

1 pound lean ground beef top round
1 teaspoon seasoning salt, like Lawry's
½ teaspoon Italian seasoning
½ teaspoon freshly ground black pepper
4 small red potatoes, unpeeled and thinly sliced
¾ cup sliced celery
1 onion, sliced
1 large red bell pepper, sliced
One 15-ounce can Italian-style chopped tomatoes, undrained
½ cup shredded reduced-fat mozzarella cheese

Preheat oven to 350°F.

In a large ovenproof skillet, cook the beef over medium heat until crumbly and just barely pink, breaking up the meat with a spoon. Drain off any excess fat.

Sprinkle the beef with the seasoning salt, Italian seasoning, and pepper. Layer the potatoes, celery, onion, and red pepper over the beef. Pour the tomatoes evenly over the top.

Cover and bake until the potatoes are tender, about 40 minutes.

Preheat the broiler.

Sprinkle the cheese evenly over the vegetables and broil until the cheese is bubbly and lightly browned, about 2 minutes. Serve in the skillet, scooping out portions with a spatula or large spoon.

Patti's Pointers: Be sure to use lean ground round, not ground beef (which is much higher in fat). Ground round will probably cost a little more, but it's up to 97 percent lean and, for my money, just as juicy and flavorful as ground beef.

If your skillet isn't ovenproof (if it has plastic handles), wrap the handles in a double layer of heavy-duty foil before putting it in the oven.

Per Serving: 180 calories, 24 g protein, 8 g carbohydrate, 5 g fat, 2.5 g saturated fat, 55 mg cholesterol, 1 g dietary fiber, 360 mg sodium

Diet Exchanges: 3 very lean meats, 1 vegetable, or ½ carbohydrate choice

For Real Veal Meat Loaf

You've heard of Sunday-go-to-meeting clothes? Well this is Sunday-go-to-eating meat loaf. It's tender, moist, and has a wickedly delicious crunchy crust. Serve it with rice and the roasted asparagus on page 154 for a menu that's hard to beat.

Makes 8 servings

One 10¾-ounce can condensed reduced-fat cream of mushroom soup
1 egg, slightly beaten
1 small bunch green onions, chopped (about ½ cup)
½ cup dry Italian-seasoned bread crumbs
1 tablespoon chopped fresh thyme or ½ teaspoon dried
¾ teaspoon salt
½ teaspoon ground black pepper
2 pounds ground veal

Preheat the oven to 375°F. Line a baking sheet with parchment paper or foil.

In a large bowl, mix together the soup, egg, onions, bread crumbs, thyme, salt, and pepper. Using your hands, gently mix in the veal just until combined. Scrape onto the prepared pan and shape with your hands into an oblong loaf, about 12 inches long and 5 inches wide.

Bake until the veal loaf is slightly browned on the surface and no longer pink in the center, about 1 hour and 15 minutes.

Patti's Pointers: The secret to tender meat loaf is handling the meat very little. That's why it's added at the very end here, after all the other ingredients have been combined. The slightly crunchy crust takes this dish over the rainbow. To get the most out of this delicious crust, I like to bake the loaf on an open baking sheet rather than in the traditional loaf pan or casserole dish.

Per Serving: 180 calories, 19 g protein, 9 g carbohydrate, 7 g fat, 3 g saturated fat, 100 mg cholesterol, less than 1 g dietary fiber, 570 mg sodium

Diet Exchanges: 3 lean meats or ½ carbohydrate choice

Sooo Good Swiss Steak

Makes 4 servings

1 pound lean boneless beef round steak, trimmed of fat and cut into 6 pieces
¼ teaspoon ground black pepper
1 large onion, thinly sliced
½ cup sliced celery
½ cup baby carrots, sliced into coins
1 tablespoon fresh chopped thyme or ½ teaspoon dried
One 14.5-ounce can Italian-style stewed tomatoes, undrained
One 12-ounce jar beef gravy
1 tablespoon cornstarch
¼ cup water

Coat a large skillet with fat-free cooking spray and heat over medium-high heat until smoking hot. Sprinkle the beef with the pepper. Add to the pan and cook until browned all over, 1 to 2 minutes per side. Transfer the beef to a plate.

Drain any excess fat from the pan. Reduce the heat to medium and add the onion, celery, and carrots. Cook until tender, about 4 minutes.

Put the meat and juices over the vegetables. Sprinkle with the thyme. Pour the tomatoes and gravy over the top. Reduce the heat to low, cover, and cook until the meat is fork-tender, about 1 hour and 15 minutes.

Remove the meat to a platter or plates. Skim any excess fat from the gravy in the pan (there may not be much if your beef was well trimmed).

In a cup, dissolve the cornstarch in the water. Stir into the gravy in the pan and increase the heat to medium. Cook until thickened and bubbly, 1 to 2 minutes. Spoon over the beef before serving.

Patti's Pointers: If you're starting out with frozen beef, be safe and thaw it in the refrigerator instead of on your countertop. You'll reduce the risk of contamination and give the ice crystals time to be reabsorbed into the meat, creating moister beef. Thaw the beef on a tray in your refrigerator to catch any drips. For each pound of steak, allow about 3 to 5 hours thawing time.

Per Serving: 260 calories, 31 g protein, 17 g carbohydrate, 6 g fat, 3 g saturated fat, 75 mg cholesterol, 2 g dietary fiber, 780 mg sodium

Diet Exchanges: 3 very lean meats, 1 vegetable, or 1 carbohydrate choice

Melt-in-Your-Mouth Roast Tenderloin

Let me say this from the start: This dish is pricey. (A whole tenderloin runs from about $40 to $80!) That's why, at my house, it's strictly a special-occasion meal. But when you've got something truly wonderful to celebrate—a marriage, a graduation, the birth of a baby—this dish screams special.

Makes 14 servings

¼ cup olive oil
1 tablespoon Worcestershire sauce
2 tablespoons chopped fresh parsley
1 tablespoon chopped fresh rosemary
2 garlic cloves, minced
1 teaspoon salt
1 teaspoon freshly ground black pepper
1 whole beef tenderloin (4 to 5 pounds), trimmed of fat

Place the beef in a large baking dish or roasting pan (about 4-quart size).

In a medium bowl, mix together the oil, Worcestershire sauce, parsley, rosemary, garlic, salt, and pepper. Pour the mixture over the beef, thoroughly rubbing it into the meat. Cover and refrigerate for at least 1 hour, or up to 8 hours for more flavor.

Remove the beef from the refrigerator and bring it to room temperature, covered, about 1 hour before roasting.

Preheat the oven to 450°F.

Pat the beef dry and set it on a rack in a large roasting pan. Tuck under the thin end if it is much thinner than the thick end. Roast until an instant-read thermometer inserted in the thickest portion registers 135°F for medium-rare, 20 to

30 minutes. (Check the temperature often, as it climbs quickly and it would be a crime to overcook a nice—expensive!—piece of meat like this.)

Remove the roast to a platter and let it stand 10 minutes before cutting into ½-inch-thick slices.

Option: This tastes divine with low-fat Italian vinaigrette. Or to make a simple sauce from the pan drippings, skim the fat (if any) from the drippings in the roasting pan. Add 1½ cups dry red wine or low-sodium beef broth, any leftover marinade, and any juices that accumulate on the platter as the roast rests. Boil over medium-high heat, stirring and scraping the bottom of the pan until the liquid is reduced by about half. Season with ¼ teaspoon each salt and pepper (and about 2 teaspoons chopped fresh rosemary and/or parsley if you have any leftover). Serve with the roast.

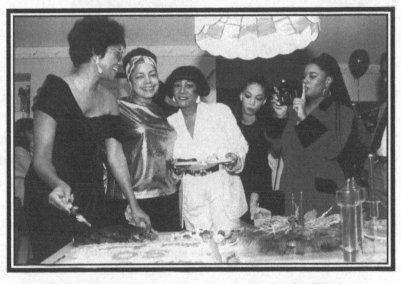

Celebrating a truly special occasion—my cousin Hazel's fiftieth birthday—with friends and family.

If you have leftovers for a few days, slice them thinly, toss with Italian vinaigrette, and serve with your favorite greens for a roast beef salad.

Per Serving: 320 calories, 38 g protein, 0 g carbohydrate, 17 g fat, 7 g saturated fat, 110 mg cholesterol, 0 g dietary fiber, 260 mg sodium

Diet Exchanges: 5 medium-fat meats or 0 carbohydrate choices

Lamb Chops LaBelle

When my sister-friend and coauthor, Laura Randolph Lancaster, got married a few years ago, she served lamb chops at her wedding reception. Now, I'm not a fan of hotel food (that's putting it mildly; I usually hate it), but I have to give whoever cooked these lamb chops their props. They were off-the-hook delicious. They were so good, in fact, that when I went home I started working on my own recipe for Lamb Chops La-Belle. It took me more than a few times to get the recipe just right, especially since I wanted to do the chops lite and right. Lite is a big deal to Laura; several people she is close to have diabetes. She is always bugging me about what I'm eating, if I'm exercising, whether I'm taking my medicine and checking my sugar. I won't lie: Sometimes the child gets on my last good nerve with all her questions. So on her wedding day I decided it was my turn to get on *her* nerves. (Don't roll your eyes; turnabout is fair play.) I knew that Laura was planning to wear a pair of pumps that had—and I am being very generous here—a two-inch heel *at best*. If I'm lying, I'm flying. The first time she showed them to me, I had a fit.

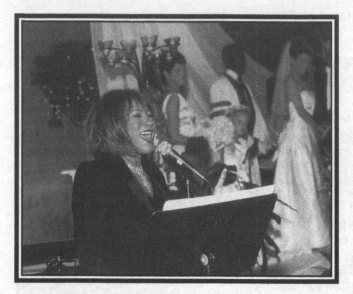

Singing at Laura's wedding—*after* she agreed to wear the pumps! (Photo by Roosevelt Sharpe)

"No you're not wearing those old lady shoes when you get married," I told her. "I don't know any grandmothers who would be caught dead wearing those things in church on Sunday morning, let alone walking down the aisle in them on their wedding night."

Laura tried to win my sympathy. "Pat, be reasonable. I'm going to be on my feet all night long. Don't you want me to be comfortable?"

I don't know why she thought I was going to let the subject drop. Of all people, she knows that I'm the same way about pumps as I am about pans. They have to be right. No half-stepping. Not long after that conversation I called my friend the super talented designer Donna Karan, and you know what I asked for: a pair of her fabulous pumps. In Laura's size. In the exact shade of her wedding dress. I have to say Miss Donna outdid herself. The shoes—a pair of white satin mules—were dazzling. Sexy. To-die-for gorgeous. Best of all, the heels were five inches!

The morning of Laura's wedding I took them out of my suitcase and handed them to her. "Here," I said in my best I-am-not-playing-with-you voice. "You're wearing these."

Long pause. "Pat, they're absolutely beautiful but I can't wear them. The heel is too high. We've been all through this."

Longer pause. "You want me to sing, right?" I said.

"Yes."

"Well, I want you to wear these pumps."

Both of us got what we wanted, although Laura knew I would have sung at her wedding even if she had worn the grandmother pumps. The wedding was as beautiful as the shoes. And I got the inspiration for a luscious lamb chop recipe out of the deal to boot.

Makes 4 servings

2 tablespoons olive oil
2 tablespoons fresh lemon juice
2 tablespoons Worcestershire sauce
1 tablespoon chopped fresh rosemary
1 tablespoon chopped fresh oregano
1 tablespoon chopped fresh basil
1 garlic clove, minced
½ teaspoon salt
¼ teaspoon freshly ground black pepper
8 lamb loin chops (about 4 ounces each), trimmed of fat

In a large resealable plastic bag, combine the olive oil, lemon juice, Worcestershire sauce, rosemary, oregano, basil, garlic, salt, and pepper. Add the chops and shake to coat completely. Refrigerate for at least 1 hour, or up to 4 hours for more flavor.

Preheat the oven to 500°F.

Heat a cast-iron or other heavy ovenproof skillet over medium-high heat until smoking hot, 4 to 5 minutes. Remove the chops from the marinade and place in the pan. Immediately transfer the pan to the oven. Cook, turning once, until browned on both sides and an instant-read thermometer registers 145°F for medium-rare, 3 to 4 minutes per side. The center should still be slightly pink.

Patti's Pointers: If your kitchen has good ventilation, you can brown these chops completely on the stove top instead of finishing them in the oven. But you'll get a lot less smoke if you pop them in the oven. Or you could preheat the pan in the oven and skip preheating on the stove top. But I find that the direct heat of the stove top heats the pan quicker and makes it hotter, giving you a better sear on the meat. When shopping for your lamb chops, for fat- and flavor-conscious cooking, look for the words "loin" or "leg." These cuts tend to be the leanest and the tastiest.

Per Serving: 430 calories, 34 g protein, 1 g carbohydrate, 31 g fat, 14 g saturated fat, 135 mg cholesterol, 0 g dietary fiber, 260 mg sodium

Diet Exchanges: 5 medium-fat meats, 3 fats, or 0 carbohydrate choices

Burnin' Beef Stroganoff

When shopping for beef, here's what you have to remember: The leanest cuts have the words "round" or "loin" in them. Eye of round, top round, sirloin, and tenderloin are some examples. Besides being lean, *tender*loin really lives up to its name—for my money it's the tenderest cut you can buy. Cooked whole, like the recipe on page 88, it makes a drop-dead dramatic entrée for company dinners. And it makes this dish virtually melt in your mouth.

Makes 6 servings

12 ounces no-yolk egg noodles
1 teaspoon reduced-calorie margarine
12 ounces beef tenderloin, trimmed of fat and cut into strips or bite-size pieces
1 onion, halved and sliced
One 14½-ounce can fat-free beef broth, divided
4 ounces mushrooms, sliced
1 teaspoon paprika
½ teaspoon Worcestershire sauce
¼ teaspoon salt
½ teaspoon ground black pepper
⅓ cup reduced-fat sour cream
1 tablespoon chopped fresh tarragon or ½ teaspoon dried

Cook the noodles according to the package instructions, leaving out any butter or salt. Drain and set aside.

Melt 1 teaspoon of the margarine in a large skillet over medium heat. Add the beef and cook, stirring frequently, until browned all over, about 5 minutes. Transfer the beef to a plate, leaving the juices in the pan.

Add the onion to the pan and cook until tender, about 5 minutes.

Raise the heat to medium-high, add half of the broth, and cook 10 minutes more.

Add the mushrooms, paprika, Worcestershire sauce, salt, and pepper. Cook, stirring, until most of the liquid has evaporated, 8 to 10 minutes.

Stir in the beef, remaining half of the broth, sour cream, and tarragon. Cook until heated through, about 2 minutes.

Toss the noodles with about ¼ cup of the beef sauce to moisten. Serve the beef mixture over the noodles.

Patti's Pointers: When choosing beef, look for meat with a cherry-red color. And if you see lots of liquid in the package, leave it right there in the meat case. That usually means it's been frozen and thawed. And, if you don't want to pay $10 or $12 per pound for beef tenderloin, go for extra-lean stew beef instead. It's often cut from the very lean top round and only costs about $3.50 per pound. If you can find Angus beef, grab it. It will be even *more* tender because it comes from a younger animal.

Per Serving: 350 calories, 18 g protein, 43 g carbohydrate, 11 g fat, 4.5 g saturated fat, 85 mg cholesterol, 2 g dietary fiber, 290 mg sodium

Diet Exchanges: 2 lean meats, 3 starches, 1 fat, or 3 carbohydrate choices

Down-Home Pork Chops in Guilt-Free Gravy

Comfort food at its finest. Need I say more?

Makes 4 servings

4 boneless center-cut loin pork chops (about 4 ounces each)
2 cups chopped onions
1 garlic clove, minced
1 cup fat-free reduced-sodium beef broth
1 teaspoon seasoning salt, such as Lawry's
¼ teaspoon white or black pepper
2 tablespoons cornstarch
⅓ cup fat-free half-and-half
1 tablespoon chopped fresh rosemary (optional)

Coat a large skillet with fat-free cooking spray and heat over medium-high heat until smoking hot.

Add the chops and cook until browned on both sides, 2 to 3 minutes per side. Transfer the chops to a plate.

Reduce the heat to medium and add the onions and garlic to the skillet. Cook until tender, about 4 minutes.

Stir in the broth, seasoning salt, and pepper. Return the chops to the skillet. Reduce the heat to low, cover, cook until the chops register 160°F on an instant-read thermometer and the juices run clear, 10 to 12 minutes.

Meanwhile, dissolve the cornstarch in the half-and-half. Pour into the skillet and cook, stirring constantly, until the gravy thickens, 2 to 3 minutes more.

Per Serving: 180 calories, 22 g protein, 9 g carbohydrate, 6 g fat, 2 g saturated fat, 55 mg cholesterol, 1 g dietary fiber, 420 mg sodium

Diet Exchanges: 3 lean meats, 1 vegetable, or ½ carbohydrate choice

Patti's Potato and Ham Frittata

On those days when the clock says it's time for dinner but your taste buds say it's time for breakfast, this dish will hit the spot.

Makes 4 servings

¼ cup chopped red pepper
¼ cup chopped green onions
2 cups frozen hash-brown potatoes
½ cup chopped cooked ham
1½ cups fat-free egg substitute, such as Egg Beaters
2 tablespoons chopped fresh tarragon or parsley or 1 teaspoon dried
2 tablespoons fat-free half-and-half
½ teaspoon salt
¼ teaspoon white or black pepper
¼ cup shredded reduced-fat cheddar cheese

Coat an ovenproof skillet with fat-free cooking spray and heat over medium heat. Add the red pepper and green onions and cook until tender, about 4 minutes. Add the potatoes, cover, and cook 10 minutes more, stirring often.

Stir in the ham and cook until heated through, about 2 minutes.

In a medium bowl, whisk together the egg substitute, tarragon or parsley, half-and-half, salt, and white or black pepper. Set aside.

Preheat the broiler. Pour the egg mixture into the skillet and cook, stirring occasionally to let the uncooked egg reach the bottom of the pan. Cook until the bottom is set and the top is still somewhat loose, 5 to 8 minutes.

Sprinkle with the cheese and run the skillet under the broiler until puffy and the cheese is lightly golden, 1 to 2 minutes.

Option: Use whatever ham you like in this dish: Chopped ham steak, chopped canned ham, or even reduced-fat breakfast sausage all work well. If using breakfast sausage, cook it in the same pan you plan to use for the frittata.

Per Serving: 240 calories, 22 g protein, 21 g carbohydrate, 7 g fat, 2.5 g saturated fat, 20 mg cholesterol, 2 g dietary fiber, 520 mg sodium

Diet Exchanges: 3 medium-fat meats, 1½ starches, or 1½ carbohydrate choices

Righteous Rump Roast

My aunt Hattie Mae makes a rump roast that is out of this world. I don't know what she does to it but the meat just melts in your mouth. Melt-in-your-mouth delicious is just what I was going for here. And if I do say so myself, I think Aunt Hattie would be proud.

Makes 12 servings

1 teaspoon paprika
1½ teaspoons salt
½ teaspoon ground black pepper
½ teaspoon garlic powder
One 4-pound lean rump roast, trimmed
½ cup fat-free beef broth
10 small whole white boiler onions, peeled
4 celery ribs, chopped
1 cup sliced fresh mushrooms
Two 8-ounce cans reduced-sodium tomato sauce
¾ cups reduced-fat sour cream
2 tablespoons chopped fresh parsley

Mix the paprika, salt, pepper, and garlic powder on waxed paper or a cutting board. Roll the roast in the seasoning and rub into the meat to coat completely.

Coat a Dutch oven with fat-free cooking spray and heat over medium-high heat until smoking hot. Add the roast and cook until browned all over, 1 to 2 minutes per side.

Reduce the heat to medium-low and pour in the broth. Cover and simmer for 1 hour and 30 minutes.

Skim off any excess fat from the surface of the liquid in the pan. Halve the onions lengthwise if they are large. Scatter the onions, celery, and mushrooms around the roast. Pour in the tomato sauce, cover, and simmer until the vegetables are tender and the meat registers 160°F on an instant-read thermometer, 45 to 55 minutes. Stir in the sour cream and parsley.

Patti's Pointers: If you can't find a 4-pound rump roast, bottom round roast works just as well.

Per Serving: 310 calories, 33 g protein, 7 g carbohydrate, 17 g fat, 7 g saturated fat, 105 mg cholesterol, 1 g dietary fiber, 390 mg sodium

Diet Exchanges: 4 medium-fat meats, 1 vegetable, or ½ carbohydrate choice

"Barbecue" Pork Chops

You know the saying "sing for your supper"? Well, one night I did just that. I wanted to cook these pork chops for Sunday dinner but the market where I buy my meats closed a few minutes before I got there. I could see folks inside closing up so I just knocked on the window and, well, you know the famous Temptations song "Ain't Too Proud to Beg"? Enough said. One of the employees took pity on me and unlocked the door. I was pretty sure he didn't recognize me because I had on my disguise—big sunglasses and an even bigger hat. But my high-heeled pumps gave me away. (I don't do flat shoes, even when I'm trying to be anonymous.) Boyfriend looked at them, then he looked at me. He looked at me, then he looked at them.

"Oh my God," he whispered, "you're Patti LaBelle."

"Yeah, Sugar, it's me," I said, trying to get my chops and get out of there fast, quick, and in a hurry. "Don't tell anybody. And thanks for letting me in."

You can pretty much guess where this story is headed.

"Miss LaBelle," he said as he was ringing up my chops, "I'm a big fan. A *really* big fan. Before you leave, would you mind singing just a little something?"

What could I say? The kid *had* let me in after closing time. So, right there at the cash register, I crooned a few bars of "When You've Been Blessed, Pass It On." I thought that was the right note to leave on, don't you?

Makes 6 servings

6 boneless center-cut loin pork chops, about 4 ounces each
½ cup fat-free low-sodium chicken broth or water, divided
¼ cup reduced-fat Caesar dressing (not creamy)
¼ cup light teriyaki sauce, such as Kikkoman's
¼ cup chili sauce
2 teaspoons brown sugar replacement, such as Brown Sugar Twin
½ teaspoon poultry seasoning
1 tablespoon cornstarch

Coat a large skillet with fat-free cooking spray and heat over medium-high heat until smoking hot. Add the chops and cook until browned on both sides, 2 to 3 minutes per side. Drain off any excess fat.

In a medium bowl, combine ¼ cup of the broth or water, the Caesar dressing, teriyaki sauce, chili sauce, brown sugar replacement, and poultry seasoning. Reduce the heat to medium-low and pour the mixture over the chops. Cover and simmer for 20 minutes.

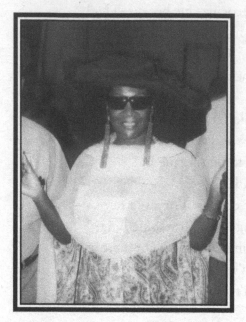

Yours truly in disguise—or so I thought!

Turn the chops over and cook, covered, until the chops register 160°F on an instant-read thermometer, about 20 to 25 minutes more.

Dissolve the cornstarch in the remaining ¼ cup of broth or water. Move the chops to the side and pour the cornstarch mixture into the skillet. Cook, stirring constantly, until the sauce thickens, 1 to 2 minutes.

Per Serving: 200 calories, 26 g protein, 5 g carbohydrate, 8 g fat, 2.5 g saturated fat, 75 mg cholesterol, 0 g dietary fiber, 430 mg sodium

Diet Exchanges: 3 medium-fat meats or 0 carbohydrate choices

Pass-It-On Pork Crown Roast

Early in my career, when my son Zuri was small, I missed a lot of special times with him and my family. Times I'll never get back—birthdays, holidays, Mom-will-you-come-see-my-school-play days. In the seventies, Labelle was trying to break into the big leagues and we were out on the road a lot. Even the most *special* holidays were no exception, although I know now that they should have been. Years ago my best friend, Claudette, tried to tell me how important it was to spend them with friends and family.

"Patsy, please," she pleaded one long-ago November afternoon. "You have to come home for Thanksgiving this year."

I told Claudette what I always did. "This tour is too important, maybe next year."

There aren't many decisions I've made in my life that I've regretted more. Since that phone call from Claudette, I've been out on hundreds of tours. But that was the last holiday I ever had the chance to celebrate with Claudette. Shortly after, my sister-in-spirit died of breast cancer at the age of thirty-eight.

I'll never forget what Claudette said when I told her I couldn't come home. I only wish I'd listened to what she said.

"Friends and family should always come first, Patsy. They don't read your résumé at your funeral."

This is a friends-and-family recipe. The kind of meal you serve when you're celebrating something special—like being home for the holidays. And good friends like Claudette.

Makes 14 servings

1 tablespoon olive oil
1 garlic clove, minced
1 teaspoon poultry seasoning
1 teaspoon salt, divided
¾ teaspoon ground black pepper, divided
1 pork rib crown roast (5 to 6 pounds, 12 to 14 ribs)
1 onion, quartered
1 cup baby carrots
1 celery rib, sliced
½ cup water or more, as needed
1½ cups dry white wine

Preheat the oven to 450°F.

In a cup, mix together the olive oil, garlic, poultry seasoning, ¾ teaspoon of the salt, and ½ teaspoon of the pepper. Thoroughly rub the roast with this mixture, making sure to rub the meat of each rib.

Place the roast on a rack in a roasting pan. Wrap a small piece of foil around the tips of each of the rib bones to prevent blackening (see Patti's Pointers). Scatter the onion, carrots, and celery around the roast. Roast for 20 minutes.

Reduce the heat to 325°F and drizzle ¼ cup of the water over the vegetables. Roast until the meat registers 150°F on an instant read thermometer (without touching bone), about 1 hour and 45 minutes more. Drizzle the vegetables with more water, ¼ cup at a time, whenever they begin to look dry (which will depend upon the amount of fat on your roast). Transfer the roast to a platter and let stand 10 minutes before serving.

Transfer the vegetables to a strainer and skim the fat from the pan juices (see Patti's Pointers). Hold the strainer over the roasting pan and press the vegetables with a potato masher to squeeze as much juice as possible from the vegetables into the pan.

Place the roasting pan over one or two burners on medium-high heat and pour in the wine. Boil until the liquid is reduced by half. Stir in the remaining ¼ teaspoon salt and ¼ teaspoon pepper. Serve the pan sauce with the roast.

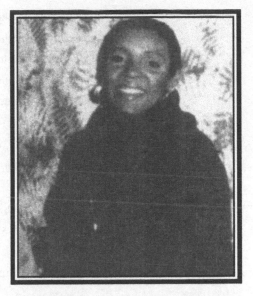

The beautiful and beloved Claudette, my sister-in-spirit.

Option: This roast looks even more impressive served with stuffing in the center. Cook your favorite stuffing in a separate baking dish in the oven along with the roast (you'll need 5 to 6 cups stuffing, enough to fill an 8-inch-square pan). Spoon the cooked stuffing into the center of the roast before serving. Want the over-the-top look without the over-the-top calories? Fill the center with a whole head of roasted cauliflower or your favorite prepared side dish vegetable.

Patti's Pointers: Like the Melt-in-Your-Mouth Roast Tenderloin on page 88, this dish is a real dazzler. We're talking fall-down-on-the-floor-and-weep flavor and appearance. That said, at my house, it's another strictly special-occasion meal. Make that *super* special occasion. (You'll know why when the butcher hands you the bill.) Price, I'm sure, is one good reason I have yet to find a pork crown roast in the meat case at the supermarket. So remember, when you're ready to prepare this dish, you'll have to order it in advance from your butcher.

To make those cute little decorative foil covers for the bones, cut twelve to fourteen 3-inch-square pieces of foil (cut the same number of pieces as rib bones on your roast). Wrap each piece of foil around the butt end of a carrot to create a rounded top. Slip a formed piece of foil over each rib bone and pinch the bottom of the foil securely onto the bone, leaving the top puffed and rounded. All that cutting and wrapping too much hassle? Then just wrap the bones in foil to prevent blackening. Before serving, remove them and top the bones with pitted olives, paper frills (sold in most grocery stores)—or with no topping whatsoever.

Here's another great timesaving secret: To de-fat the pan juices, use a fat separator. It looks like a plastic measuring cup with a spout that reaches to the bottom of the cup. The fat rises to the top of the cup—then you just pour out the pan juices through the bottom spout. *Brilliant.*

And last but not least, to carve the roast easily, insert a fork in the top of the roast to steady it and make downward slices close to each rib bone.

Per Serving: 320 calories, 28 g protein, 2 g carbohydrate, 20 g fat, 7 g saturated fat, 85 mg cholesterol, less than 1 g dietary fiber, 390 mg sodium

Diet Exchanges: 4 medium-fat meats or 0 carbohydrate choices

People-Pleasing Poultry

Terrific Turkey Pasta Casserole

Makes 6 servings

6 ounces wide no-yolk egg noodles
1 tablespoon margarine
1 cup chopped celery
1 cup sliced mushrooms
½ cup chopped red bell pepper
½ cup chopped green onions, including green part
1½ pounds 95 percent lean ground turkey (not 99 percent lean turkey breast; see headnote on Serious Sloppy Joes, page 28)
One 10¾-ounce can 98 percent fat-free condensed cream of mushroom soup
2 tablespoons light teriyaki sauce, such as Kikkoman
1½ teaspoons poultry seasoning
½ teaspoon salt
½ teaspoon ground black pepper
¼ teaspoon red pepper flakes
8 ounces reduced-fat sour cream
¼ teaspoon paprika

Preheat the oven to 325°F. Coat a 2-quart baking dish with fat-free cooking spray.

Cook the noodles according to package instructions, leaving out any salt or butter. Drain and set aside.

Meanwhile, melt the margarine in a large saucepan over medium heat. Add the celery, mushrooms, red bell pepper, and green onions. Cook until just tender, about 4 minutes. Add the turkey and cook, breaking up the meat with a spoon, until the turkey is no longer pink, about 5 minutes. Drain off any excess liquid.

Stir in the soup, teriyaki sauce, poultry seasoning, salt, black pepper, and red pepper flakes. Bring to a boil over high heat. Reduce the heat to low, cover, and simmer for 15 minutes, stirring often.

Stir in the sour cream and noodles. Pour the mixture into the prepared baking dish and sprinkle with the paprika. Cover with foil, and bake until heated through, about 15 minutes.

Patti's Pointers: Be sure and use *light* teriyaki sauce; the regular kind has goo-gobs of sodium. With all the other goodies in this dish, I promise you won't miss the taste. And if you're trying to shake the salt habit, use only 1 tablespoon of the teriyaki sauce. Before digging in, you can season with your favorite salt substitute if needed.

Per Serving: 330 calories, 25 g protein, 21 g carbohydrate, 16 g fat, 6 g saturated fat, 115 mg cholesterol, 2 g dietary fiber, 710 mg sodium

Diet Exchanges: 3 lean meats, 1 fat, 1 vegetable, or 1½ carbohydrate choices

Really Good Roast Chicken Caesar

When I was a kid, I spent the summers with my Grandmother Ellen on her farm in Florida. Grandmother Ellen believed in chicken eating but she didn't believe in chicken buying. At least not from a store. When Grandmother Ellen felt like cooking chicken, she'd just go outside, choose a nice fat bird, then swing it over her head until she broke its neck. In no time she'd have it cleaned, plucked, and fried. And it was so good it would put the Colonel's to shame. While Grandmother Ellen wouldn't be caught dead buying or baking a chicken, you can do both. The results will be seriously delicious, not to mention a whole lot easier on you—and the chicken.

Makes 6 servings

One 3½- to 4-pound chicken (with skin)
1 lemon, pierced all over with a fork
4 garlic cloves, smashed
½ cup lite Caesar dressing (not creamy), such as Ken's Steakhouse
2 teaspoons rotisserie chicken seasoning, such as McCormick's
1 teaspoon poultry seasoning
1 teaspoon Italian seasoning
½ teaspoon ground black pepper
¼ teaspoon red pepper flakes

Preheat the oven to 450°F.

Rinse the chicken and chicken cavity in cold water and pat dry inside and out with paper towels.

Put the lemon and garlic inside the chicken cavity.

In a small bowl, mix together the Caesar dressing, rotisserie chicken seasoning, poultry seasoning, Italian seasoning, black pepper, and red pepper flakes. Brush the mixture all over the chicken.

Place the chicken breast side down on a rack in a roasting pan; roast for 20 minutes.

Reduce the heat to 350°F. Turn the chicken breast side up on the rack and brush all over with the seasoning mixture. Roast, brushing with the seasoning mixture two more times, until an instant-read thermometer registers 165°F when inserted into a thigh and the juices run clear, 35 to 40 minutes more.

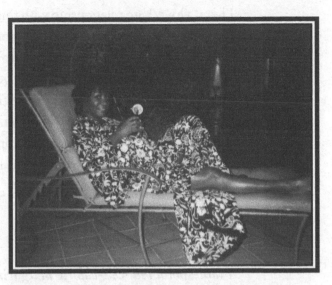

At home chilling poolside until my chicken gets done. (That's water, not soda, in the glass!)

Remove from the oven and let rest for 5 minutes before serving.

Patti's Pointers: I use rotisserie chicken seasoning instead of plain table salt in this recipe because it gives the chicken that gorgeous golden-brown color home ovens rarely produce but commercially cooked rotisserie chicken is famous for. To reduce the fat and calories even more, remove the skin before eating. The chicken will be so moist and flavorful you won't even miss it.

To turn the hot chicken during cooking, remove the chicken from the oven and stick the handles of two long wooden spoons into both ends of the bird. Rotate the chicken on the handles to turn over.

Per Serving: 510 calories, 42 g protein, 6 g carbohydrate, 35 g fat, 10 g saturated fat, 205 mg cholesterol, 0 g dietary fiber, 580 mg sodium

Diet Exchanges: 6 lean meats, 3 fats, or ½ carbohydrate choice

Chicken Cacciatore

I have a love/hate relationship with this recipe. I love it because it's a family-filling favorite. I hate it because it fills the house with such heavenly aromas that, whenever I cook it, everybody crowds into my kitchen. We'll be packed in there like sardines and nobody will offer to leave. When you make this dish at your house, the same thing is sure to happen. When it does, use my Grandmother Ellen's surefire way of getting everybody out. Grab a pan—Grandmother Ellen always used a big old cast-iron skillet—and, in your best I-am-not-joking voice, tell folks that if they're not gone when you finish counting to ten you're going to hit somebody upside the head with it.

Makes 6 servings

1 tablespoon reduced-calorie margarine
3 medium yellow squash, halved lengthwise and thinly sliced
1 large onion, thinly sliced
1 large green pepper, cut into strips
¾ cup sliced fresh mushrooms
One 14.5-ounce can Italian-style stewed tomatoes, undrained
1 tablespoon chopped fresh oregano or 1 teaspoon dried
1 tablespoon chopped fresh parsley or 1 teaspoon dried
1 teaspoon poultry seasoning
½ teaspoon freshly ground black pepper
Six 4-ounce boneless, skinless chicken breasts
⅓ cup grated Parmesan cheese
½ teaspoon paprika

Preheat the oven to 375°F.

Melt the margarine in a large, deep ovenproof sauté pan or stove-top casserole dish over medium heat. Add the squash, onion, green pepper, mushrooms, tomatoes, oregano, parsley, poultry seasoning, and black pepper. Bring to a boil over high heat. Reduce the heat to low, cover, and simmer until the vegetables are tender, about 10 minutes.

Arrange the chicken on top of the vegetables. Sprinkle with the Parmesan and paprika. Cover and bake until an instant-read thermometer registers 160°F in a breast and the juices run clear, 25 to 30 minutes.

Turn on the broiler and broil until the top is nicely browned, about 5 minutes.

Option: This dish is wonderful over pasta. And rice works well, too. Either way, you'll need ½ cup uncooked for each serving (3 cups total).

Patti's Pointers: If you have a deep skillet with plastic handles, you can still use it. Just wrap the handles in several layers of heavy-duty foil to protect them while the skillet is in the oven.

Per Serving: 260 calories, 34 g protein, 14 g carbohydrate, 7 g fat, 2.5 g saturated fat, 85 mg cholesterol, 4 g dietary fiber, 350 mg sodium

Diet Exchanges: 4 very lean meats, 2 vegetables, 1 fat, or 1 carbohydrate choice

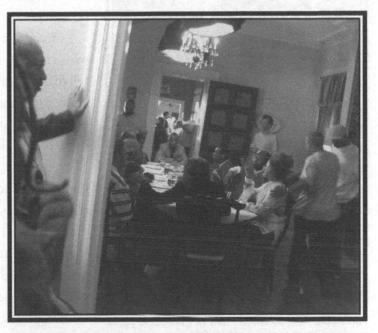

Too many folks for me to count crowding in the dining room after I kicked them out of the kitchen.

Sensational Skewers

Before my sisters got sick, every summer we'd throw a barbecue in Chubby's backyard and invite everybody we knew. Ask anyone who ever came to one: Those barbecues were all-the-way live. I don't know which was longer, the guest list or the grocery list, but both were gigantic. We told people to come early (to eat) and stay late (to party). When it came to the menu, moderation was not a concept the Holte sisters were into. The night before the barbecue, none of us slept. We stayed up all night long getting everything ready—marinating this, chopping that, spicing and slicing and dicing enough food to feed the whole neighborhood and half of Philly. Between the four of us, we made so many dishes we had to set up five or six picnic tables just to hold them all. If I close my eyes, I can still see the spread: the chicken and the chops, the collards and the coleslaw, the corn and the casseroles and the cobblers. It wasn't just a barbecue; it was a banquet.

Every now and then, I'll run into someone who came to those barbecues, and they always tell me the same thing: Every one of them was an affair to remember. Every one of them was barbecue bliss. And not just because of the food, although if I do say so myself, it was smokin'. Literally and figuratively. While the food was slamming, people still remember those barbecues all these years later because of the feeling in the space, the joy in the place. My older sister, Vivian, used to say that the best barbecues happened on nights when the moon was full. She said that's when the stars sprinkled magic dust. Looking back on those barbecues, I know one thing for certain and two things for sure: There *was* magic at them. But it came from Vivian, not

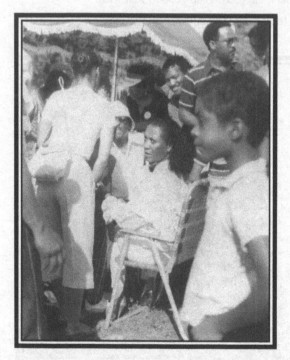

The whole neighborhood, half of Philly, and yours truly at one of those magical, memory-making barbecues. That's my son, Zuri, in the foreground. Wasn't he an adorable little kid?

the stars. Once folks finished eating (their first plate at least), the party was on. We'd crank up the stereo and dance and sing and tell tall tales until the wee hours of the morning. Vivian loved herself some blues. And when she played them, nobody was allowed to sit down. Nobody. She'd throw on some B.B. King or Bobby "Blue" Bland and go around the yard until she'd gotten everybody out of their chair and out on the floor—or I should say out on the grass. It was a blast. The stuff memories are made of.

At your next barbecue, I want you to do me a favor. Two favors, actually. First, add these wonderful skewers to your menu. When cooked over medium-high coals, they take on that nothing-like-it-in-the-world-cooked-over-charcoal flavor and that heavenly grilled aroma. Then, when the cookout is in full swing, throw on some B.B. King. Let him play "Lucille"—*loud*—just like Vivian used to. I can't make any promises but, if the moon is full and the food is right, you just might channel her spirit into your backyard. You'll know it worked if you feel the magic dust.

Makes 6 servings

2 ears corn, each cut into 8 equal pieces
⅔ cup fat-free Italian vinaigrette dressing (not creamy)
1 tablespoon chopped fresh basil
1 tablespoon chopped fresh cilantro
1 teaspoon poultry seasoning
½ teaspoon salt
½ teaspoon ground black pepper
1½ pounds boneless, skinless chicken breasts, cut into 1-inch pieces
1 large sweet onion (such as Vidalia), halved and cut into wedges
1 large green bell pepper, cut into 1-inch pieces
1 pint cherry tomatoes

In a large microwave-safe dish, microwave the corn on high for 3 minutes. Set aside.

In a large bowl, combine the vinaigrette, basil, cilantro, poultry seasoning, salt, and pepper. Add the corn, chicken pieces, onion, green pepper, and cherry tomatoes. Cover and marinate in the refrigerator for at least 1 hour, or up to 4 hours, stirring occasionally.

Preheat the grill to medium or turn on the broiler. Remove the chicken from the marinade and drain; discard the marinade.

Put the chicken, onion, bell pepper, corn, and tomatoes on skewers, alternating the ingredients in that order.

Grill or broil 4 inches from the heat until the chicken is no longer pink in the center, 5 to 8 minutes.

Patti's Pointers: To ensure even grilling, cut all of your ingredients into the same size pieces and turn the skewers once during grilling. I use metal skewers, preferably the two-pronged kind, because your meat and vegetables won't move around when you're turning them and they don't burn or splinter, as wooden ones can. (See the skewers on the cover.) If you are using wooden skewers, however, as my friends in the islands would say, "no problem." Just be sure to soak them in cold water for half an hour before putting your skewer together; this usually keeps them from charring during grilling. And if you're up for a little extra work, work that—I promise—will take your skewers to a whole new level, try this little trick: soak wooden skewers in fresh lemon juice for 30 minutes. Don't ask me why, but the lemon juice gives the skewers a fly-you-to-the-moon flavor that will have folks talking about them until next year's barbecue.

In addition to metal skewers, you'll need a good sturdy knife such as a cleaver to cut the corn into pieces or "wheels." Set the cob on a cutting board and cut the cob crosswise into eight "wheels." For each cut, hold the cob with one hand and with the other hand push the knife down through the kernels and just into the hard inner cob. Then take your one hand off the cob and place it open on the top side of the knife and push down through the cob with all of your weight. Or, if you have an accurate strike, raise the cleaver one to two feet above the corn cob and quickly and accurately bring it down onto and through the cob for each cut.

Per Serving: 200 calories, 24 g protein, 17 g carbohydrate, 4.5 g fat, 1 g saturated fat, 55 mg cholesterol, 3 g dietary fiber, 125 mg sodium

Diet Exchanges: 3 very lean meats, 1 starch, 1 vegetable, or 1 carbohydrate choice

Oven (Tastes Like Southern) Fried Chicken

I created this recipe in honor of my late sister-friend the legendary singer-songwriter Laura Nyro. The day I met Laura I knew we were going to be lifelong friends. Laura was the real deal. Talented (I used to tell her she could sing like a sister). Kind as she could be. A brilliant artist (everybody from Frank Sinatra to Aretha Franklin has recorded her songs). Had loads of money but none of the I'm-all-that-and-a-bag-of-chips attitude that often goes with it. Just a real cool woman. Every time I was going through a crisis, every time I was facing a crucial crossroads in my life, Laura was there for me. Back in the seventies, for example, when creative differences between Sarah, Nona, and me started to tear Labelle apart, it was Laura who told me the time had come for me to leave.

"Just walk away, Pat," she said. "In the long run it will be better for everyone."

When I told Laura I couldn't, not because I didn't want to but because I was scared—scared of hurting Sarah and Nona, scared of letting down my fans, scared that I couldn't make it on my own—she gave me some of the best advice I've ever heard.

"Pat," she said, "many a false step is made by standing still."

I didn't know what she meant at the time. But decades later, when my marriage was coming apart and I stayed in it long after I should have left, Laura's words came back to me. And I finally understood.

Laura was a fan of my fried chicken and potato salad the way I was a fan of her music. For years, she tried everything to get me to give her those two recipes. Everything from begging ("Please, Pat, I won't tell another soul") to bribing ("I'll take you to the seafood market and you can buy the place out").

When Laura fell in love and got married, I gave her my potato salad recipe as a wedding gift. But I never gave her the one for fried chicken. I can only hope she would have loved this recipe as much as the original. And as much as I loved her.

Makes 4 servings

1 teaspoon salt
1 cup warm water
Four 4-ounce boneless, skinless chicken breasts
1 egg
½ cup fat-free buttermilk
1½ cups plain dry bread crumbs
1 teaspoon poultry seasoning
1 teaspoon freshly ground black pepper
½ teaspoon salt
¼ teaspoon seasoning salt, such as Lawry's
⅛ teaspoon ground red pepper

In a large bowl, dissolve the salt in the water. Add the chicken and enough cold water to cover the chicken. Cover and refrigerate for at least 3 hours, or up to 6 hours.

Preheat the oven to 450°F. Line a baking sheet with aluminum foil and coat the foil with fat-free cooking spray. Drain the chicken and pat dry.

In a large bowl, whisk together the egg and buttermilk.

In a large resealable plastic bag, mix together the bread crumbs, poultry seasoning, black pepper, salt, seasoning salt, and red pepper.

Dip the chicken, one breast at a time, in the buttermilk mixture, then place in the bag with the bread-crumb mixture. Shake well to coat, then transfer to a rack. Repeat with remaining chicken breasts.

Put the baking sheet in the oven until smoking hot, about 2 minutes.

Coat both sides of the chicken with fat-free cooking spray and place on the hot baking sheet. Bake until an instant-read thermometer registers 160°F in a breast and the juices run clear, about 30 to 35 minutes.

Turn on the broiler and broil 4 inches from the heat to brown the top, about 5 minutes.

Patti's Pointers: While I know it's tempting to skip the chicken-soaking part, don't! Soaking the chicken seals in the moisture and prevents the chicken from drying out during cooking. The result: that juicy-on-the-inside, crunchy-on-the-outside taste that the great Southern cooks in my family were famous for. Try it, and don't be surprised if the Colonel calls you for *your* recipe!

Per Serving: 310 calories, 34 g protein, 31 g carbohydrate, 5 g fat, 1.5 g saturated fat, 115 mg cholesterol, 1 g dietary fiber, 850 mg sodium

Diet Exchanges: 3 very lean meats, 2 starches, or 2 carbohydrate choices

Easy-as-Pie Honey Mustard Chicken Thighs

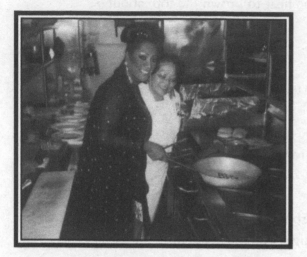

Hanging out in a fabulous hotel kitchen with its first lady, Miss Ming, after a show.

I like to prepare this dish when I'm out on the road because it's super easy to make. Brush and bake; that's all there is to it! While I always try to book a hotel suite with a kitchen, sometimes that's just not possible. Sometimes, not often but sometimes, if I'm kitchenless and my electric frying pans won't do, I'll talk somebody into letting me use the hotel's. I've been in some that are just too fabulous. A cook's dream. Huge. High-tech. Home to all kinds of culinary wonders. Everything from state-of-the-art appliances to simply spectacular spices. The last time I cooked in a hotel kitchen, I made these chicken thighs because I didn't want to be in the way and I could get in and out in half an hour. But if you cook them at home they'll be just as good.

Makes 4 servings

¼ cup honey
¼ cup country-style Dijon mustard
1 tablespoon chili sauce
1 teaspoon mustard seed
½ teaspoon mustard powder
½ teaspoon salt
½ teaspoon ground black pepper
¼ teaspoon garlic powder
8 boneless, skinless chicken thighs (about 1¼ pounds), trimmed of fat

In a medium bowl, mix together the honey, mustard, chili sauce, mustard seed, mustard powder, salt, black pepper, and garlic powder. Add the chicken, turning to coat. Cover and marinate in the refrigerator for at least 1 hour, or up to 6 hours.

Preheat the oven to 375°F.

Coat a shallow roasting pan with fat-free cooking spray. Arrange the chicken in a single layer in the pan. Cover with foil and bake for 30 minutes.

Turn the chicken over and brush with any remaining honey-mustard mixture. Bake, uncovered, until the chicken is no longer pink in the center and the juices run clear, 20 to 25 minutes more.

Per Serving: 220 calories, 24 g protein, 19 g carbohydrate, 6 g fat, 1 g saturated fat, 0 g dietary fiber, 95 mg cholesterol, 620 mg sodium

Diet Exchanges: 3 very lean meats, 1 starch, 1 fat, or 1 carbohydrate choice

Superb Seven-Spice Chicken Breasts

Here's a great quick-baked dish for busy nights.

Makes 6 servings

1½ teaspoons Chinese five-spice powder
1 teaspoon paprika
1 teaspoon curry powder
½ teaspoon ground red pepper
½ teaspoon garlic powder
¼ teaspoon chili powder
¼ teaspoon ground turmeric
One 14.5-ounce can Mexican-style stewed tomatoes with jalapeño peppers and
*   spices, undrained*
Six 4-ounce boneless, skinless chicken breasts

Preheat the oven to 325°F. Coat a 13 × 9-inch glass baking dish with fat-free cooking spray.

In a small bowl, mix together the five-spice powder, paprika, curry powder, ground red pepper, garlic powder, chili powder, and ground turmeric.

Rub both sides of the chicken breasts with the spice mixture.

Put the chicken in the prepared pan and pour the tomatoes evenly over the top. Bake for 30 minutes.

Turn the chicken over and bake until the chicken registers 160°F on an instant-read thermometer and the juices run clear, about 30 minutes more.

Option: This dish tastes great served over curried rice.

Per Serving: 200 calories, 34 g protein, 8 g carbohydrate, 2 g fat, 0 g saturated fat, 80 mg cholesterol, 1 g dietary fiber, 280 mg sodium

Diet Exchanges: 4 very lean meats, 1 vegetable, or 0 carbohydrate choices

Curried Chicken and Rice

Makes 4 servings

1 pound boneless, skinless chicken breasts, cut into bite-size pieces
1½ cups fat-free, reduced-sodium chicken broth
One 14.5-ounce can reduced-sodium stewed tomatoes, undrained
2 teaspoons curry powder
¼ teaspoon cinnamon
¼ teaspoon ground allspice
¼ teaspoon ground red pepper
¼ teaspoon turmeric
½ teaspoon salt
1¼ cups uncooked long-grain rice

In a large saucepan, combine the chicken, broth, tomatoes, curry powder, cinnamon, allspice, ground red pepper, turmeric, and salt. Bring to a boil over high heat.

Stir in the rice, mixing well. Reduce the heat to low, cover, and simmer until the chicken is no longer pink in the center, about 20 minutes.

Patti's Pointers: When you're shopping for curry powders, remember that they vary widely in their level of spiciness—some are weak and some are wow! If you want a good, solid curry powder with a medium heat level, use Madras-style, available in small tins at the supermarket.

Per Serving: 400 calories, 27 g protein, 61 g carbohydrate, 5 g fat, 1.5 g saturated fat, 50 mg cholesterol, 3 g dietary fiber, 570 mg sodium

Diet Exchanges: 3 very lean meats, 3 starches, 2 vegetables, or 3 carbohydrate choices

We Be Jammin' Jamaican Jerk Chicken

Spicy-hot chili pepper lovers like me know that "jerk chicken" is synonymous with "hot chicken." And I don't mean one-drop-of-Tabasco-sauce hot, either. I mean fire-breathing, five-alarm, clear-out-your-sinuses-and-make-your-nostrils-flair hot. None of that wimpy stuff for genuine, bona fide, *real* chili heads like me. This dish is my version of Jamaica's time-honored technique of "jerking" meat. To be sure that the recipe will live up to its name, when you're preparing it, do what I do: Put on some Bob Marley and get your groove on.

Makes 4 servings

2 tablespoons fresh lime juice
2 tablespoons low-sodium soy sauce
2 tablespoons jerk seasoning, such as McCormick's
1 tablespoon peanut oil or other vegetable oil
1 tablespoon Dijon mustard
1 tablespoon chopped fresh thyme
¼ cup chopped scallions or onions
2 teaspoons chopped fresh ginger
½ teaspoon poultry seasoning
¼ teaspoon ground black pepper
¼ teaspoon ground red pepper (or more to taste)
Four 4-ounce boneless, skinless chicken breasts

In a shallow baking dish, combine the lime juice, soy sauce, jerk seasoning, oil, mustard, thyme, scallions or onions, ginger, poultry seasoning, ground black pepper, and ground red pepper. Add the chicken, turning to coat completely. Cover and marinate in the refrigerator for at least 4 hours, or up to 2 days.

Coat a grill rack with fat-free cooking spray and preheat the grill to medium. Grill the chicken, turning once, until it registers 160°F on an instant-read thermometer and the juices run clear, 5 to 8 minutes per side.

Option: This dish is excellent over dirty rice or with red beans and rice.

Patti's Pointers: If you don't want to fire up the grill, you can broil the chicken instead. Coat a broiler rack with fat-free cooking spray and preheat the broiler. Broil the chicken on the rack in a broiling pan 4 to 6 inches from the heat and cook as directed.

Per Serving: 140 calories, 21 g protein, 3 g carbohydrate, 5 g fat, 1 g saturated fat, 50 mg cholesterol, 0 g dietary fiber, 710 mg sodium

Diet Exchanges: 3 very lean meats, 1 fat, or 0 carbohydrate choices

Good-as-It-Gets Grilled Chicken
with Mango Salsa

This recipe, like the recipes for Perfect Piecrust (page 192) and Marvelous Minted Snap Peas (page 162), was given to me by the talented recipe developer and cookbook author David Joachim. Grilled chicken with mango salsa makes a dramatic entrée at summer barbecues where *everybody* cooks hot dogs and hamburgers on the grill. At your next cookout, why not dazzle your guests with David's dish? And don't be mad at me when they start begging you for the recipe.

Makes 4 servings

¼ cup orange juice, divided
3 tablespoons fresh lime juice, divided
2 tablespoons extra-virgin olive oil
5 tablespoons finely chopped red onion, divided
¾ teaspoon salt, divided
¼ teaspoon ground black pepper
Four 6-ounce boneless, skinless chicken breast halves
1 mango, pitted, peeled, and finely chopped
⅛ teaspoon hot pepper sauce
1 tablespoon chopped fresh cilantro or basil

In a medium bowl, stir together 2 tablespoons of the orange juice, 2 tablespoons of the lime juice, the oil, 2 tablespoons of the onions, ½ teaspoon of the salt, and the pepper. Add the chicken, turning to coat. Cover and refrigerate for at least 1 hour, or up to 4 hours.

In another medium bowl, combine the mango, 2 tablespoons reserved orange juice, 1 tablespoon reserved lime juice, 3 tablespoons reserved onion, ¼ teaspoon reserved salt, and the hot pepper sauce. Stir in the cilantro or basil.

Coat a grill rack with fat-free cooking spray. Preheat the grill to medium. Grill the chicken 4 inches from the heat, basting occasionally with the marinade and turning once, until an instant-read thermometer registers 160°F in the thickest part and the juices run clear, 3 to 4 minutes per side. Serve with the salsa.

Patti's Pointers: To easily pit and peel a mango, stand it upright on a cutting board and slice off each flat side, curving the knife around the inner pit to remove as much flesh as possible. Lay the center pitted piece flat on the board and cut the flesh from the pit. Slice off the peel. Double up a kitchen towel in your hand and place one mango half in it. Score the flesh all the way down to the peel in a cross-hatch pattern (be careful not to cut all the way through the peel). Push up the peel side in the center to expose the cubes of flesh. Cut the flesh away from the peel. Repeat with the other mango half.

Per Serving: 210 calories, 33 g protein, 13 g carbohydrate, 3 g fat, 0.5 g saturated fat, 80 mg cholesterol, 1 g dietary fiber, 240 mg sodium

Diet Exchanges: 4 very lean meats, 1 fruit, or 1 carbohydrate choice

Tender-as-a-Love-Song Turkey Tenderloins
with Rice and Country Gravy

Turkey breast tenderloins make this dish better than good. They make it *mad* good, as the teenagers say. Because they come from the tenderest section of the turkey breast, they're so moist they almost melt in your mouth, Hungry yet?

Makes 6 servings

1½ pounds turkey tenderloins, cut into 1-inch pieces
1 teaspoon poultry seasoning
4 teaspoons margarine, divided
1 onion, chopped
2 celery stalks, chopped
1 clove garlic, minced
One 6.9-ounce box reduced-sodium rice mix, such as Rice-A-Roni
One 10¾-ounce can reduced-fat condensed cream of mushroom soup
½ cup fat-free half-and-half
1 tablespoon chopped fresh thyme or 1 teaspoon dried
¼ teaspoon ground black pepper

Season the turkey with the poultry seasoning.

Melt 2 teaspoons of the margarine in a large deep skillet. Add the onion, celery, garlic, and turkey. Cook until the vegetables are tender and the turkey is just slightly pink in the center, about 10 minutes.

Remove the turkey mixture to a plate and cover to keep warm. In the same pan, prepare the rice according to the package directions, using the remaining 2 teaspoons margarine. Spoon the turkey mixture over the rice.

In a medium bowl, whisk together the soup, half-and-half, thyme, and pepper. Pour over the turkey. Cover and cook over low heat until heated through, about 10 minutes.

Patti's Pointers: If you can't find turkey tenderloins, turkey breast cutlets or turkey breast chops will work, too.

Per Serving: 290 calories, 28 g protein, 31 g carbohydrate, 5 g fat, 1 g saturated fat, 65 mg cholesterol, 1 g dietary fiber, 900 mg sodium

Diet Exchanges: 3 very lean meats, 1 fat, 1 starch, or 1 carbohydrate choice

Tastes-Just-Like-Mom-Used-to-Make-It Chicken Pot Pie

Makes 8 servings

1 pound skinless chicken tenders
1 teaspoon poultry seasoning
½ teaspoon salt
¼ teaspoon black pepper
2 teaspoons margarine
1 onion, chopped
3 celery ribs, chopped
1 large green pepper, chopped
1 cup baby carrots, slivered
1 cup frozen green beans
One 12-ounce jar homestyle chicken gravy, such as Heinz
½ cup fat-free sour cream
2 tablespoons flour
Two 9-inch frozen piecrusts or unbaked Perfect Piecrusts (page 192)

Preheat the oven to 425°F.

Season the chicken tenders with the poultry seasoning, salt, and pepper.

Melt 1 teaspoon of the margarine in a large deep skillet or saucepan over medium heat. Add the chicken and cook just until slightly pink in the center, about 5 minutes. Remove to a cutting board. When cool, chop into bite-size pieces.

Meanwhile, melt the remaining 1 teaspoon margarine in the same skillet or saucepan. Add the onion, celery, green pepper, and carrots. Cook until the vegetables are tender, about 5 minutes. Stir in the frozen green beans and chopped chicken.

In a medium bowl, mix together the gravy, sour cream, and flour.

Stir into the chicken mixture in the skillet or saucepan.

Scrape the filling into the prepared piecrust. Carefully fit the top crust over the filling. Cut 3 to 5 slits in the top crust for ventilation.

Bake until the filling is bubbly and the crust is golden brown, 25 to 30 minutes. Let sit for 5 minutes before serving.

Patti's Pointers: Look for bottled gravies near the other bottled sauces in your supermarket. Heinz makes a line of flavored chicken gravies, such as roasted garlic, which add even more zip to this recipe.

Per Serving: 320 calories, 14 g protein, 29 g carbohydrate, 16 g fat, 4.5 g saturated fat, 25 mg cholesterol, 2 g dietary fiber, 640 mg sodium

Diet Exchanges: 1 very lean meat, 1 starch, ½ vegetable, 3 fats, or 2 carbohydrate choices

Wicked Wild Rice and Chicken Casserole

Makes 6 servings

1½ pounds boneless, skinless chicken breasts
2 teaspoons poultry seasoning
1 teaspoon ground black pepper
½ teaspoon salt
¼ teaspoon red pepper flakes
8 ounces sliced mushrooms
One 6-ounce box quick-cooking long grain and wild rice mix,
    such as Uncle Ben's
⅓ cup light Caesar dressing (not creamy)
One 16-ounce container reduced-fat sour cream, divided
1 teaspoon dried thyme

Preheat the oven to 325°F.

Season the chicken with the poultry seasoning, black pepper, salt, and red pepper flakes. Coat a large, deep, ovenproof sauté pan with fat-free cooking spray and heat over medium heat. Add the chicken and cook until no longer pink in the center, 4 to 5 minutes per side. Remove to a cutting board. When cool, chop into bite-size pieces.

Meanwhile, in the same pan, cook the mushrooms until almost tender, about 5 minutes. Remove to a bowl.

In the same pan, cook the rice according to the package directions, leaving out the butter. Stir in the mushrooms, Caesar dressing, 12 ounces (about 1½ cups) of the sour cream, the thyme, and the chopped chicken.

Bake, uncovered, until heated through, about 15 minutes. Serve with dollops of the remaining 4 ounces sour cream on each serving.

Patti's Pointers: If you don't have a large ovenproof sauté pan, cook the chicken in a wide saucepan (in batches if necessary), then use the same pan to cook the rice. When all of the ingredients have been added, transfer the mixture to a 2½-quart casserole and bake as directed.

Per Serving: 350 calories, 35 g protein, 31 g carbohydrate, 8 g fat, 5 g saturated fat, 90 mg cholesterol, 1 g dietary fiber, 930 mg sodium

Diet Exchanges: 3 very lean meats, 2 starches, 1 fat, or 2 carbohydrate choices

Chicken with Black-Eyed Peas and Yellow Rice

When you've got a soul food craving, this is the recipe to satisfy it.

Makes 6 servings

1 tablespoon olive oil
1 red onion, chopped
2 garlic cloves, minced
1½ pounds skinless chicken tenders
One 14.5-ounce can reduced-sodium chicken broth
½ teaspoon poultry seasoning
½ teaspoon ground black pepper
¼ teaspoon red pepper flakes
¼ teaspoon salt
¾ cup uncooked yellow rice (see Patti's Pointers)
One 15-ounce can black-eyed peas, drained
1 tablespoon chopped fresh thyme

Warm the olive oil in a large skillet over medium heat. Add the onions and cook until soft, about 4 minutes. Add the garlic and chicken and cook until the chicken is browned on both sides, about 4 minutes more.

Stir in the broth, poultry seasoning, black pepper, red pepper flakes, and salt. Bring mixture to a boil over high heat.

Stir in the rice. Reduce the heat to low, cover, and cook until the rice is almost tender, about 10 minutes.

Stir in the black-eyed peas and thyme. Cover and cook until heated through, about 10 minutes.

Patti's Pointers: You can find yellow rice (made with saffron) near the rice mixes in your grocery store. Look for a brand, such as Carolina, that combines the seasonings and the rice to make it easier to measure out the ¾ cup needed for this recipe. If the brand you buy comes with a separate seasoning packet, such as Goya, mix the seasonings with the rice in a separate bowl and measure out ¾ cup.

Per Serving: 300 calories, 32 g protein, 30 g carbohydrate, 5 g fat, 1 g saturated fat, 65 mg cholesterol, 3 g dietary fiber, 610 mg sodium

Diet Exchanges: 3 very lean meats, 2 starches, 1 fat, or 2 carbohydrate choices

Chicken Florentine Supreme

Here's a great light version of a classic dish.

Makes 6 servings

One 10-ounce package frozen chopped spinach
Four 4-ounce boneless, skinless chicken breasts
1 teaspoon salt
1 teaspoon poultry seasoning
1 tablespoon margarine
2 tablespoons cornstarch
1½ cups fat-free half-and-half
½ cup shredded reduced-fat Swiss cheese
¼ teaspoon ground black pepper
⅛ teaspoon grated nutmeg
¼ teaspoon paprika

Preheat the oven to 350°F. Coat a 13 × 9-inch baking dish with fat-free cooking spray.

Cook the spinach according to the package directions, leaving out any salt. Drain well.

Sprinkle the chicken all over with ¾ teaspoon of the salt and the poultry seasoning. Place the chicken breasts in the prepared pan. Arrange the spinach over and around the chicken.

Melt the margarine in a medium saucepan over medium heat. In a medium bowl, whisk together the cornstarch and half-and-half, then whisk the mixture into the margarine. Cook, whisking constantly, until the mixture bubbles and thickens.

Remove from the heat and stir in the Swiss cheese, black pepper, nutmeg, and remaining ¼ teaspoon salt until the cheese is melted.

Spoon the sauce evenly over the chicken and sprinkle with the paprika. Bake until an instant-read thermometer registers 160°F in a breast and the juices run clear, 25 to 30 minutes.

Patti's Pointers: Jarlsberg Lite makes a wonderful substitute for Swiss cheese. Look for it in blocks in the refrigerated cheese case of the dairy section of your grocery store.

Per Serving: 150 calories, 19 g protein, 6 g carbohydrate, 5 g fat, 2 g saturated fat, 40 mg cholesterol, 1 g dietary fiber, 540 sodium

Diet Exchanges: 2 lean meats, 1 vegetable, or ½ carbohydrate choice

Chicken Drumsticks
with Horseradish Sauce

Makes 6 servings

CHICKEN DRUMSTICKS

6 skinless chicken drumsticks
1½ teaspoons poultry seasoning
¾ teaspoon seasoning salt, such as Lawry's
½ teaspoon onion powder
½ cup reduced-sodium chicken broth

HORSERADISH SAUCE

½ cup reduced-fat sour cream
2 tablespoons fat-free half-and-half
2 to 3 tablespoons prepared horseradish
¼ teaspoon salt
¼ teaspoon ground black pepper

To make the chicken drumsticks: Sprinkle the chicken evenly with the poultry seasoning, seasoning salt, and onion powder.

Coat a large skillet with fat-free cooking spray and heat over medium heat. Add the chicken. Cook, turning often, until browned on all sides, about 10 minutes. Drain any excess fat.

Pour the chicken broth into the skillet and heat until boiling. Reduce the heat to medium-low, cover, and simmer until an instant-read thermometer registers 170°F in the thickest part of a drumstick (be careful not to touch bone when testing), 25 to 35 minutes.

To make the horseradish sauce: In a medium bowl, mix together the sour cream, half-and-half, 2 tablespoons of the horseradish, the salt, and the pepper. Taste and add more horseradish if desired. Serve with the drumsticks.

Patti's Pointers: If you only find skin-on drumsticks at the store, it's easy enough to skin them at home. Peel back the skin from the thick end, pulling the skin down firmly off the skinny end as if removing a sock.

Per Serving: 110 calories, 14 g protein, 3 g carbohydrate, 4.5 g fat, 2 g saturated fat, 50 mg cholesterol, 0 g dietary fiber, 340 mg sodium

Diet Exchanges: 2 lean meats, 1 fat, or 0 carbohydrate choices

Chicken Parmesan

Makes 4 servings

1 tablespoon olive oil
1 teaspoon poultry seasoning
1 teaspoon Italian seasoning
1 teaspoon garlic powder
½ teaspoon salt
3 tablespoons Italian-seasoned dry bread crumbs
2 tablespoons grated Parmesan cheese
Four 5-ounce boneless, skinless chicken breasts
1½ cups no-sugar-added tomato-basil pasta sauce, warmed
1 tablespoon chopped fresh basil

Preheat the oven to 425°F. Coat a 3-quart baking dish with fat-free cooking spray.

In a small bowl, mix together the olive oil, poultry seasoning, Italian seasoning, garlic powder, and salt. Brush the mixture evenly over the chicken.

In a shallow bowl, mix together the bread crumbs and Parmesan.

Roll the chicken breasts in the bread-crumb mixture. Place in the prepared pan and coat the top of the chicken with fat-free cooking spray.

Bake until an instant-read thermometer registers 160°F in a breast and the juices run clear, 25 to 30 minutes.

Serve with the sauce and top with the basil.

Option: This dish is a natural on a bed of linguine. Figure on 5 cups total cooked. A sprinkling of Parmesan is the final touch!

Per Serving: 290 calories, 32 g protein, 11 g carbohydrate, 12 g fat, 3 g saturated fat, 90 mg cholesterol, 1 g dietary fiber, 580 mg sodium

Diet Exchanges: 4 very lean meats, 1 fat, or 1 carbohydrate choice

Heavenly Herb-baked Chicken and Mushroom Casserole

My adopted aunt Naomi is the inspiration for this recipe. She could make a mean casserole. But what used to trip me out is that she could make it with anything in the house—*anything*. Aunt Naomi didn't believe in wasting food. "Child, that cost good money," she would say if she caught me throwing out so much as an onion skin. As long as it hadn't spoiled, Aunt Naomi didn't throw out food. She did, however, put all kinds of it into her casseroles. She would reach in the refrigerator and pull out some bits of this and some pieces of that, reach in the cabinet and beat in some of this and blend in some of that. Then she'd season it, sample it, and stir it all together. "I'm not eating any of that," I would tell her after I'd watched her make it. "I don't even think you know what's in it." Do you know how many times I had to eat my words so that Aunt Naomi would let me eat her casseroles? Every single time. She died not long ago but she'll live in my heart forever.

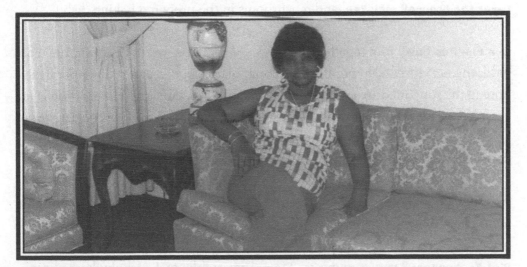

My adopted Aunt Naomi. I called her famous casseroles "refrigerator casseroles" because that's what she made them with—everything in the refrigerator.

Makes 6 servings

One 14-ounce bag frozen broccoli florets
One 12.5-ounce can chunk white chicken in water, drained
One 6-ounce jar sliced mushrooms, drained
One 10¾-ounce can reduced-fat condensed cream of mushroom soup
¾ cup reduced-fat mayonnaise, such as Hellmann's Just 2 Good!
¾ cup reduced-sodium chicken broth or water
1 tablespoon chopped fresh oregano
1 tablespoon chopped fresh basil
1 tablespoon chopped fresh thyme
1 tablespoon chopped fresh chives
¼ teaspoon salt
½ teaspoon poultry seasoning
½ teaspoon ground black pepper
¼ teaspoon red pepper flakes
3 tablespoons Italian-seasoned dry bread crumbs

Preheat the oven to 350°F. Coat a 1½-quart baking dish with fat-free cooking spray.

Layer the broccoli, chicken, and mushrooms in the prepared baking dish.

In a medium bowl, mix together the soup, mayonnaise, broth or water, oregano, basil, thyme, chives, salt, poultry seasoning, black pepper, and red pepper flakes. Spread the soup mixture evenly over the mushrooms, chicken, and broccoli layer. Sprinkle evenly with the bread crumbs. Coat the top with fat-free cooking spray.

Cover with foil and bake until heated through, about 25 minutes.

Per Serving: 260 calories, 23 g protein, 15 g carbohydrate, 12 g fat, 3 g saturated fat, 60 mg cholesterol, 3 g dietary fiber, 880 mg sodium

Diet Exchanges: 2 very lean meats, 2 fats, 1 vegetable, or 1 carbohydrate choice

Turkey and Broccoli Fettuccine in Herb Cream Sauce

Make 6 servings

8 ounces dried fettuccine noodles
4 cups broccoli florets (about 1 large head broccoli)
4 boneless, skinless turkey breast cutlets (about 1 pound)
1 teaspoon salt
1 teaspoon poultry seasoning
½ teaspoon freshly ground black pepper
8 ounces reduced-fat ricotta cheese
½ cup fat-free half-and-half
⅓ cup grated Parmesan cheese
¼ teaspoon red pepper flakes
1 tablespoon chopped fresh oregano or 1 teaspoon dried
1 tablespoon chopped fresh basil or 1 teaspoon dried

Cook the noodles according to the package directions, leaving out any butter or salt. Add the broccoli to the pasta water during the last 5 minutes of cooking. Drain and return the mixture to the pasta pot.

Meanwhile, sprinkle the turkey with ½ teaspoon of the salt, ½ teaspoon of the poultry seasoning, and ¼ teaspoon of the black pepper.

Coat a large deep skillet with fat-free cooking spray and heat over medium heat. Add the turkey and cook until no longer pink in the center, 2 to 3 minutes per side. Remove to a cutting board. When cool, cut into bite-size pieces.

In the same saucepan used to cook the turkey, combine the ricotta cheese, half-and-half, Parmesan cheese, red pepper flakes, oregano, basil, remaining ½ teaspoon salt, remaining ½ teaspoon poultry seasoning, and remaining ¼ teaspoon black pepper. Cook over medium-low heat, stirring frequently, until the sauce thickens slightly, about 8 minutes. Stir in the cooked chopped turkey breast and cook for 5 minutes.

Add a small amount of the sauce to the pasta and broccoli mixture and toss to moisten. Divide the pasta mixture among 6 plates and top with the turkey mixture.

Per Serving: 310 calories, 34 g protein, 31 g carbohydrate, 7 g fat, 3.5 g saturated fat, 65 mg cholesterol, 5 g dietary fiber, 710 mg sodium

Diet Exchanges: 3 very lean meats, 1 fat, 1 starch, 2 vegetables, or 2 carbohydrate choices

Scrumptious Sides

Stove Top Sweet Potatoes

My mother was famous all over Philly for her candied sweet potatoes. During holiday season, our phone would ring off the hook with friends and neighbors calling to ask Chubby to make her signature dish for their Thanksgiving and Christmas dinner. While, for me, nothing will ever match Chubby's recipe, this one comes pretty close.

Makes 4 servings

1 tablespoon margarine
1½ pounds sweet potatoes, peeled and cut into bite-size pieces
2 tablespoons brown sugar replacement, like Brown Sugar Twin
½ teaspoon salt
¼ teaspoon ground black pepper
¼ teaspoon ground allspice
¼ teaspoon grated nutmeg

Melt the margarine in a large skillet over medium-low heat. Add the sweet potatoes, cover, and cook, stirring occasionally, until tender, 15 to 20 minutes.

Stir in the brown sugar replacement, salt, pepper, allspice, and nutmeg. Cook 2 minutes more. Serve warm.

Patti's Pointers: Sweet potatoes are loaded with health-boosting beta-carotene. To get the most beta for your buck, shop for sweet potatoes with rich orange flesh. The darker the flesh the more beta-carotene you'll get. Also, have a little fat with your meal to help your body absorb this fat-soluble nutrient. The small amount of margarine in this recipe is just the right amount.

Per Serving: 200 calories, 3 g protein, 40 g carbohydrate, 3 g fat, 0.5 g saturated fat, 0 mg cholesterol, 4 g dietary fiber, 340 mg sodium

Diet Exchanges: 1 fat, 2 starches, or 2½ carbohydrate choices

Zesty Zucchini Casserole

Makes 8 servings

1 tablespoon margarine
1 small red onion, chopped
1 cup chopped celery
2 pounds zucchini (about 4 medium), halved lengthwise and sliced
½ teaspoon salt
½ teaspoon dried thyme
¼ teaspoon red pepper flakes
¼ teaspoon ground white or black pepper
2 tablespoons cornstarch
½ cup fat-free half-and-half
½ cup reduced-fat sour cream
¼ cup shredded reduced-fat sharp cheddar cheese, divided
½ cup plain dry bread crumbs

Preheat the oven to 350°F.

Melt the margarine in a large skillet over medium heat. Add the onion and celery and cook, stirring often, until tender, about 5 minutes. Add the zucchini, salt, thyme, red pepper flakes, and pepper. Cook until the zucchini is just tender, 8 to 10 minutes.

In a cup, dissolve the cornstarch in the half-and-half. Pour over the zucchini and cook, stirring, until thickened and coating the vegetables, about 2 minutes.

Remove from the heat and stir in the sour cream and 3 tablespoons of the cheese. Scrape into a 2-quart baking dish. Mix together the bread crumbs and remaining tablespoon of cheese. Sprinkle evenly over the top.

Bake until bubbly, about 20 minutes. Turn on the broiler and broil until the top is lightly browned, about 1 minute.

Patti's Pointers: If you ever have leftover fresh zucchini, here's another easy way to serve it. Fire up the grill and cut the zucchini lengthwise into slabs about ½ inch thick. Brush both sides of the slabs with a mixture of olive oil, salt, and pepper. Grill over a medium-hot fire until tender, 3 to 5 minutes per side. Serve as whole slabs (great in sandwiches too!) or cut into bite-size pieces and serve as a side dish. Absolutely delicious and sooooo simple.

Per Serving: 100 calories, 5 g protein, 13 g carbohydrate, 3.5 g fat, 1.5 g saturated fat, 5 mg cholesterol, 2 g dietary fiber, 280 mg sodium

Diet Exchanges: 1 starch, 1 fat, or 1 carbohydrate choice

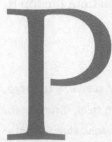**eople are always asking me why** I'm so into health-related causes. I can't tell you how many times I've heard the same question: "Patti, what's this thing you have about supporting organizations that help sick people?" And they're right. I *do* have a thing about it. You don't want to know the number of health-related organizations I've been spokesperson for: the National Cancer Institute, the National Minority AIDS Council, the National Medical Association, to name just three.

Whenever people ask me why I do it, I wish I could give some grand, high-falutin' answer. An answer that would make me sound virtuous without being self-righteous. An answer that would go something like:

I agree with whatever wise soul said that service is the rent we pay for living in this world. It is so important, so crucial, for every single one of us to do something, however small, to help those in need. I've been so blessed in my life that I can't not *give something back. Not and look at myself in the mirror in the morning.*

And while all of those things are true, the answer that comes closer to the straight-no-chaser truth is this: because, for me, the cause is personal. *Real* personal. Not some abstract mission or academic undertaking. When you lose all three of your sisters to cancer before they reach their forty-fourth birthdays, personal is the only thing it *can* be. When you have to allow doctors to amputate both your mother's legs before you lose her to complications from diabetes, how could it be anything else? When you watch Alzheimer's disease steal your daddy's mind and then take him from this world, well, I'll say it again: Personal is the only thing it can be.

"Get in where you fit in," Chubby used to say. I fit in lending my support to top-notch health-related organizations because I've lost too many people I love too many times.

Which is why, when former U. S. Health and Human Services Secretary and Morehouse School of Medicine President Emeritus Louis W. Sullivan and his lovely wife, Ginger, asked me to come to their home to say "thank you" to the many people who have supported the medical school I said, "Tell me what time to be there." The mission of the school is near and dear to my heart: "To train primary care physicians to care for people living in underserved communities." I know what you're thinking: Say what? Let me translate: The school trains people to care for poor people who live in poor places. People who, once they become doctors, will take their little black bags and set up practices in communities where other doctors won't. And you know why they won't? You get three guesses and the first two don't count. Because many of the people who live there don't have money or health insurance to pay a doctor. That, or the location is not on anybody's top-ten list of great places to live. And often both.

After I said my thank yous, I got one of the most wonderful surprises of my life. The school is building a brick courtyard/pathway to handle the traffic created by its new National Center for Primary Care. (Former Surgeon General David Satcher is heading it up.) In the courtyard and on the pathway, every single brick will bear the name of someone special. Not necessarily someone rich and famous and nationally celebrated. Someone loved. Someone prized and respected. Someone treasured. And guess whose names are going to be on the first three bricks that will be laid? My beloved sisters—Vivian, Barbara, and Jackie.

When Dr. Sullivan showed me those bricks and I saw their names on them, I couldn't hold back the tears. Several years ago, when I got my star on the Hollywood Walk of Fame, I remember thinking, *I wish my sisters could be here with me to share this moment and this honor.* Looking at those bricks, I felt like these were my sisters' stars on *their* walk of fame. And I couldn't have been prouder.

Roasted Asparagus

This dish was on the menu at the Sullivans' fabulous party. Once you taste it, you're going to be glad asparagus is available practically year round.

Makes 6 servings

2 pounds thin asparagus, trimmed
½ teaspoon salt
¼ teaspoon ground white or black pepper

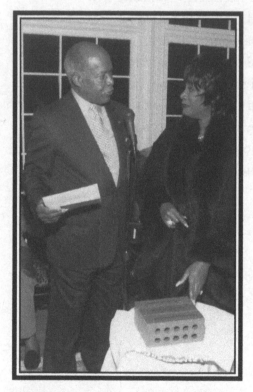

Trying to hold back tears as Dr. Sullivan presents me with the Bricks. If you look real closely you can see my sisters' names. (Photo by Horace Henry)

Preheat the oven to 450°F.

Spread the asparagus on a large baking sheet and coat with fat-free cooking spray, shaking to coat completely.

Roast until the asparagus is just tender, about 5 minutes, shaking the pan once or twice.

Sprinkle with the salt and pepper, shaking to distribute evenly.

Option: If you want to go all out, sprinkle the roasted asparagus with 1 tablespoon grated Parmesan cheese.

Patti's Pointers: To trim asparagus, hold one or two spears in your hands and bend the stalk. It will naturally break at the point where it becomes tough. If you want a touch more flavor, sprinkle the roasted asparagus with the grated zest of 1 lemon.

Per Serving: 35 calories, 4 g protein, 6 g carbohydrate, 0 g fat, 0 g saturated fat, 0 mg cholesterol, 2 g dietary fiber, 210 mg sodium

Diet Exchanges: 1 vegetable or ½ carbohydrate choice

Succotash Supreme

This makes a great side dish to the veal meat loaf on page 84.

Makes 6 servings

1 tablespoon margarine
1 small white onion, chopped
One 10-ounce package frozen lima beans
½ cup fat-free reduced-sodium chicken broth
½ teaspoon ham-flavored seasoning, such as Goya
⅛ teaspoon paprika
2 cups fresh or frozen yellow corn
2 tablespoons chopped fresh parsley

Melt the margarine in a large skillet over medium heat. Add the onion and cook until very tender, 5 to 7 minutes. Add the lima beans, broth, ham-flavored seasoning, and paprika. Reduce the heat to medium-low, cover, and cook 5 minutes.

Stir in the corn and parsley and cook until heated through, 5 to 7 minutes more.

Patti's Pointers: Fresh corn really makes this dish special (you'll need about 4 medium ears of corn). To scrape the kernels from the cob, stand the cobs upright in a shallow bowl and cut off a few rows of kernels at a time. When the kernels are removed, run the dull side of the knife down the length of the cob all the way around to extract the "milk." Add the "milk" along with the corn kernels.

Per Serving: 120 calories, 5 g protein, 22 g carbohydrate, 2.5 g fat, 0 g saturated fat, 0 mg cholesterol, 5 g dietary fiber, 130 mg sodium

Diet Exchanges: 1 starch or 1 carbohydrate choice

Simply Wonderful Squash and Sweet Onions

Makes 6 servings

1 tablespoon margarine
1 large sweet onion, such as Vidalia, sliced and separated into rings
2 pounds yellow squash, rinsed and thinly sliced
¾ teaspoon salt
½ teaspoon ground white or black pepper
2 tablespoons chopped fresh oregano and/or basil

Melt the margarine in a large deep skillet over medium heat.

Add the onion and cook until tender, about 5 minutes.

Stir in the squash, salt, and pepper. Cook until the squash is tender, about 5 minutes more. Stir in the oregano and/or basil.

Per Serving: 50 calories, 2 g protein, 8 g carbohydrate, 2 g fat, 0 g saturated fat, 0 mg cholesterol, 3 g dietary fiber, 320 mg sodium

Diet Exchanges: 2 vegetables or ½ carbohydrate choice

Sweet 'n' Spicy Baby Carrots

Thanks to the flavors of brown sugar, allspice, and nutmeg, even kids will eat these carrots.

Makes 4 servings

¼ cup fat-free reduced-sodium chicken broth
One 1-pound bag baby carrots
1 tablespoon margarine
2 tablespoons brown sugar replacement, like Brown Sugar Twin
½ teaspoon ground allspice
¼ teaspoon grated nutmeg
¼ teaspoon salt
¼ teaspoon ground black pepper

Bring the broth to a simmer in a large skillet over medium heat. Add the carrots, cover, and simmer until just tender, about 10 minutes. Stir in the margarine, brown sugar replacement, allspice, nutmeg, salt, and pepper. Cook, stirring occasionally, 2 to 3 minutes more.

Patti's Pointers: Cooking carrots for a few minutes helps to release their beta-carotene and make the nutrient more available to your body.

Per Serving: 70 calories, 1 g protein, 10 g carbohydrate, 3 g fat, 0 g saturated fat, 0 mg cholesterol, 5 g dietary fiber, 270 mg sodium

Diet Exchanges: 2 vegetables, 1 fat, or ½ carbohydrate choice

Roasted Broccoli Florets
with Garlic "Butter" Sauce

Makes 8 servings

2 pounds broccoli, cut into florets (about 8 cups)
⅓ cup plus ½ cup fat-free reduced-sodium chicken broth, divided
1 tablespoon olive oil
2 garlic cloves, minced
¼ teaspoon salt
¼ teaspoon ground white or black pepper
⅛ teaspoon red pepper flakes
One ½-ounce packet fat-free butter-flavored mix, such as Butter Buds
   (about 3 tablespoons)

Preheat the oven to 400°F.

Heat a large, deep, ovenproof skillet over medium-high heat until hot. Add the broccoli and ⅓ cup of the broth. Immediately cover the pan and cook, shaking the pan occasionally, until the broccoli is bright green and almost crisp-tender, 3 to 4 minutes. Remove from the heat and stir in the oil, garlic, salt, white or black pepper, and red pepper flakes.

Transfer the pan to the oven and roast, uncovered, until the broccoli is crisp-tender, 10 to 12 minutes.

Meanwhile, heat the remaining ½ cup broth in a microwave-safe cup until hot, 1 to 2 minutes. Dissolve the butter-flavored mix in the broth. Pour over the broccoli and toss to coat. Transfer to a serving dish if desired and serve immediately.

Patti's Pointers: If you don't have a deep ovenproof skillet (one with metal handles), cook the broccoli in a saucepan or wok, then transfer it to a shallow roasting pan. And to quickly cut a head of broccoli into florets, cut off the stalk crosswise as close to the bottom layer of florets as possible, cutting through the small stems that attach the florets to the stalk. The bottom layer of florets will fall away from the stalk. Continue making crosswise cuts across the small stems that attach the remaining layers of florets to the stalk.

Per Serving: 45 calories, 2 g protein, 6 g carbohydrate, 2 g fat, 0 g saturated fat, 0 mg cholesterol, 2 g dietary fiber, 80 mg sodium

Diet Exchanges: 1 vegetable or ½ carbohydrate choice

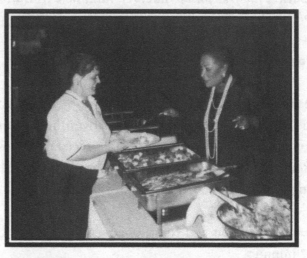

Checking out what the veggies are cooked in before digging in.

Down-Home Cabbage

The secret to melt-in-your-mouth cabbage is slow cooking; it makes it tender as a Grammy-winning love song.

Makes 8 servings

¼ cup fat-free reduced-sodium chicken broth or water
1 teaspoon ham-flavored seasoning, such as Goya
½ teaspoon salt
½ teaspoon ground white or black pepper
1 medium head green cabbage, about 2 pounds, cored and sliced

Mix the broth or water, ham-flavored seasoning, salt, and pepper in a large deep skillet or saucepan over low heat. Add the cabbage, cover, and cook, stirring occasionally, until the cabbage is tender, 45 to 55 minutes.

Patti's Pointers: To easily core and slice cabbage, peel off and discard any tough outer leaves. Using a large knife, cut the cabbage in half through the core. Cut out and discard the core from each half. Slice the cabbage crosswise into thin strips.

Per Serving: 40 calories, 2 g protein, 8 g carbohydrate, 0 g fat, 0 g saturated fat, 0 mg cholesterol, 3 g dietary fiber, 340 mg sodium

Diet Exchanges: 1 vegetable or ½ carbohydrate choice

Marvelous Minted Snap Peas

I like to make this recipe in midsummer, when snap peas are at their sweetest and snappiest. It couldn't be simpler and the flavor is sublime.

Makes 6 servings

3 tablespoons reduced-calorie margarine
1 pound sugar snap peas, strings removed
3 scallions, chopped
2 tablespoons chopped fresh mint
½ teaspoon salt
¼ teaspoon ground black pepper

Melt the margarine in a skillet over medium heat. Stir in the peas and scallions. Cover and cook until the peas are bright green and crisp-tender, 1 to 2 minutes. Stir in the mint, salt, and pepper. Serve warm.

Option: I sometimes flavor these peas a bit more by adding the grated zest of one small lemon along with the mint.

Patti's Pointers: To remove the strings from sugar snap peas, snap off the stem end sideways, then pull it down the length of the pod to remove the strings on both sides (there may be just one string on each side).

Per Serving: 100 calories, 2 g protein, 9 g carbohydrate, 6 g fat, 1 g saturated fat, 0 mg cholesterol, 3 g dietary fiber, 350 mg sodium

Diet Exchanges: 1 starch, 1 fat, or ½ carbohydrate choice

Creamed Spinach

This dish is beaucoup times better than the boil-in-a-bag versions. And, if you use bags of prewashed baby spinach, almost as easy to prepare.

Makes 6 servings

4 scallions, chopped (about 1 cup)
Three 10-ounce packages fresh baby spinach
2 tablespoons cornstarch
½ cup fat-free half-and-half
3 ounces reduced-fat cream cheese
¼ cup reduced-fat sour cream
½ cup chopped fresh chives
½ teaspoon salt
¼ teaspoon white or black pepper
⅛ teaspoon red pepper flakes

Coat a medium saucepan with fat-free cooking spray and heat over medium heat. Add the scallions and cook until tender, about 5 minutes.

Add the spinach and cook, stirring occasionally, until spinach is just wilted, about 5 minutes.

Whisk together the cornstarch and half-and-half until the cornstarch is dissolved. Move the spinach to the sides of the pan and pour the cornstarch mixture in the center. Cook and stir until thickened, about 2 to 3 minutes. Reduce the heat to low and stir in the cream cheese, sour cream, chives, salt, white or black pepper, and red pepper flakes. Cook until creamy and heated through, about 1 minute.

Patti's Pointers: Always dissolve cornstarch in cold liquid before adding it to a hot pan; otherwise you'll get lumps.

Per Serving: 100 calories, 7 g protein, 11 g carbohydrate, 4 g fat, 2.5 g saturated fat, 10 mg cholesterol, 4 g dietary fiber, 370 mg sodium

Diet Exchanges: 1 vegetable, 1 fat, or 1 carbohydrate choice

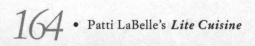

Classic Corn Pudding

Kids can't get enough of this creamy corn dish. Truth be told, neither can I.

Makes 6 servings

1 tablespoon margarine
½ cup finely chopped onion
1½ cups fat-free half-and-half
1 tablespoon cornstarch (See Patti's Pointer's on creamed spinach recipe,
    page 164)
2 cups fresh or frozen corn kernels
1 large egg, lightly beaten
1 teaspoon sugar substitute, such as DiabetiSweet or Splenda
½ teaspoon salt
¼ teaspoon ground white or black pepper
⅛ teaspoon paprika

Preheat the oven to 325°F. Coat a 1-quart baking dish with fat-free cooking spray.

Melt the margarine in a medium saucepan over medium heat. Add the onion and cook until tender, about 5 minutes.

Whisk together the half-and-half and cornstarch until the cornstarch dissolves. Pour into the pan and cook, whisking constantly, until the mixture thickens, 2 to 3 minutes. Remove from the heat and stir in the corn, egg, sugar substitute, salt, and pepper. Pour into the prepared baking dish and sprinkle with the paprika.

Bake until bubbly and set on the surface, 55 to 60 minutes.

Per Serving: 110 calories, 5 g protein, 16 g carbohydrate, 3.5 g fat, 0.5 g saturated fat, 35 mg cholesterol, 2 g dietary fiber, 260 mg sodium

Diet Exchanges: 1 starch or 1 carbohydrate choice

Good-as-It-Gets Green Bean Casserole

Makes 8 servings

1 teaspoon margarine
1 cup chopped white onion
2 garlic cloves, minced
3 cups fat-free half-and-half
¼ cup cornstarch
1 pound fresh green beans, trimmed, or one 16-ounce bag frozen green beans,
    thawed and drained
2 tablespoons chopped fresh basil
¾ teaspoon salt
¼ teaspoon ground black pepper
½ cup plain dry bread crumbs

Preheat the oven to 400°F. Coat a 3-quart baking dish with fat-free cooking spray.

Melt the margarine in a medium saucepan over medium heat. Add the onion and garlic and cook, stirring occasionally, until tender, about 5 minutes.

Whisk together the half-and-half and cornstarch until the cornstarch dissolves. Pour into the pan and whisk until thickened, 3 to 5 minutes.

Remove from the heat and stir in the green beans, basil, salt, and pepper. Spoon into the prepared baking dish and sprinkle with the bread crumbs. Bake until bubbly, 20 to 25 minutes. Turn on the broiler and broil until the crumbs are lightly browned, about 1 minute.

Patti's Pointers: To quickly trim fresh green beans, line up some of the green beans on a cutting board and cut across the stem ends with a large knife in a single cut. Repeat with the remaining green beans.

Per Serving: 100 calories, 5 g protein, 18 g carbohydrate, 1 g fat, 0 g saturated fat, 0 mg cholesterol, 2 g dietary fiber, 340 mg sodium

Diet Exchanges: 1 vegetable, 1 starch, or 1 carbohydrate choice

Delectable Vegetable Medley

Want the kids in your house to eat their vegetables? This recipe will have them asking for seconds.

Makes 6 servings

1 cup fresh broccoli florets
1 cup fresh asparagus, trimmed and cut into 2-inch lengths
1 packed cup fresh baby spinach
1 cup sliced yellow squash
⅓ cup finely chopped onions
One 10¾-ounce can reduced-fat condensed cream of mushroom soup
½ cup water
1 tablespoon chopped fresh oregano and/or basil
¼ teaspoon salt
¼ teaspoon ground black pepper

Preheat the oven to 350°F. Coat a 2-quart baking dish with fat-free cooking spray.

Layer the broccoli, asparagus, spinach, squash, and onions in the prepared baking dish.

In a small bowl, mix together the soup, water, oregano and/or basil, salt, and pepper. Pour over the vegetables. Cover with foil and bake until the broccoli is crisp-tender, 30 to 35 minutes. Uncover and serve immediately.

Patti's Pointers: Asparagus doesn't keep long so plan to use it as soon as you can. To keep it fresh in the fridge, store it stem ends down in a glass filled with a few inches of water, and cover loosely with a plastic bag. If you forget to store it this way, you can help revive limp asparagus by slicing off a bit of the stem ends, then refrigerating the asparagus stem ends down as described (but using ice water) for about 2 hours.

Per Serving: 50 calories, 3 g protein, 8 g carbohydrate, 1 g fat, 0 g saturated fat, 0 mg cholesterol, 2 g dietary fiber, 300 mg sodium

Diet Exchanges: 1 vegetable or ½ carbohydrate choice

Dreamy
Desserts

I was a daddy's girl. A *serious* one. I wish you could have known him; he was as cool as a cucumber. And fine as wine. When I was little, he spoiled me rotten. Like Chubby, he could get down in the kitchen and he knew how much I loved his cooking. Anything I wanted he'd make for me—breakfast, lunch, dinner, snacks. If I wanted it, all I had to do was ask for it. Everything Daddy cooked was fly-you-to-the-moon good, but his desserts, well, they were over the rainbow. I don't know which I craved more—Daddy's food or his love. All I know is that I ate both of them up.

Before Chubby and Daddy separated, when my sisters and I were little, every morning before school he would fix our braids and our breakfast. He made these cinnamon rolls that would make you hurt yourself. Those rolls were so good that just smelling them would make you start speaking in tongues. My sisters always complained that whenever Daddy cooked our breakfast, he always gave me the biggest helpings. Of course, Daddy would always deny it.

"You know better than that," he would say, giving us all a big hug. "I treat all my girls the same."

I don't know about the size of the helpings of his food, but I do know about the size of the helpings of Daddy's love. They were massive. Mammoth. Major. In the summer, after we'd eaten dinner, Daddy and I would sit on the front porch together and sing duets. He had a voice almost as smooth as his rap and, let me tell you, that is saying something. As the ladies who knew him will attest, Daddy's rap was serious. Sublime. So, so cool. Family legend has it that once, when he was at the Club Harlem in Atlantic City, he had half the women in the place hanging on his every word. Daddy loved to flirt. Whenever Chubby gave him the blues about it he would tell her the same thing: "Just because I'm not ordering anything doesn't mean I can't look at the menu."

But let me get back to that night at the Club Harlem. All the attention Daddy was getting made the buddy he had ridden up with so jealous that he told Daddy it was time to head back to Philly. Well, Daddy wasn't trying to hear that. Not when he had his mojo working. Not when he had it dialed up to ten. So Daddy told his buddy that he wasn't ready and he wasn't leaving. But he understood if his buddy wasn't *staying*.

"You go on back without me," he told him in his real-cool way. "I'll walk home if I have to."

And that's just what Daddy did. All the way from Atlantic City to Philly. No one knows exactly why but he ended up at the home of our neighbors, the ones who had gotten him his first job in Philly—Oliver and Florine Llockman. After he took a nap and drank a glass of water, he came on home. That story gives you a pretty good idea of the kind of man Daddy was. He lived life on his own terms. He made his own rules. And he always made a way out of no way.

He was also one of the first people in my life who made me believe that maybe, just maybe, I could really sing. Not in a pleasant-but-not-all-that-special kind of way. In a turn-the-show-out-blow-the-doors-off-the-place kind of way.

"Baby girl," he would say on those nights when we were singing our duets on the front porch. "You got the pipes. *Star* pipes. And when you become one, I'm going to be your biggest fan."

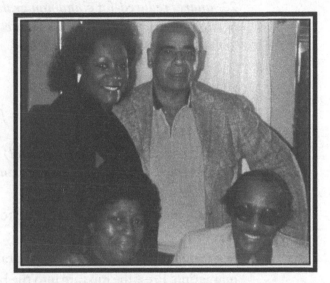

My super cool Dad, Henry Holte (wearing the shades, of course), Oliver and Florine Llockman and me back in the old neighborhood—back in the day.

And he was. Long before I was so much as a blip on the music industry's radar screen, Daddy came to all kinds of holes-in-the-wall to hear me sing. The way he would clap and cheer you would have thought I was playing Carnegie Hall instead of some tiny little town hall.

That's why I'm dedicating the dessert chapter to him. Not just one recipe. The whole chapter. Like the desserts in it, Daddy was unusually dreamy and uncommonly sweet.

Wonderful White Chocolate Pie

Makes 10 servings

CRUST

20 squares reduced-fat cinnamon graham cracker squares, crushed into crumbs
¼ cup sugar substitute, such as DiabetiSweet or Splenda
⅓ cup margarine, melted

FILLING

One 1-ounce package fat-free, sugar-free instant white chocolate pie filling
2 cups fat-free half-and-half
½ teaspoon almond extract (optional)
7 sugar-free crème-filled chocolate sandwich cookies, coarsely chopped

To make the crust: Preheat the oven to 375°F.

In a medium bowl, mix together the graham cracker crumbs, sugar substitute, and margarine. Press the mixture into the bottom and up the sides of a 9-inch pie pan.

Bake for 10 minutes. Cool on a rack.

To make the filling: In a medium bowl, using an electric mixer on medium speed, beat the pie filling mix, half-and-half, and almond extract (if using), until smooth, about 2 minutes. Stir in the chopped cookies.

Pour the filling into the crust, cover with foil, and refrigerate until set, about 3 hours.

Patti's Pointers: If you have a food processor, make the crust in it to save time. Process the graham crackers into crumbs, then add the sugar substitute. Instead of melting the margarine, cut it into pieces, add to the food processor bowl, and pulse until well mixed. For a nice touch, garnish with a sprinkle of unsweetened cocoa powder before serving.

Per Serving: 180 calories, 3 g protein, 23 g carbohydrate, 9 g fat, 1.5 g saturated fat, 0 mg cholesterol, 0 g dietary fiber, 340 mg sodium

Diet Exchanges: 1½ starches, 2 fats, or 1½ carbohydrate choices

Very Berry Trifle

When you have a crowd coming for dinner and you need a glamorous-as-it-is-delicious dessert, you can't do better than this one. It is *gorgeous*. But don't take my word for it; flip to the cover and see for yourself.

Makes 12 servings

1 recipe Four-Flavor Sour Cream Pound Cake (page 179)
One 1-ounce package fat-free, sugar-free instant vanilla pudding mix
2 cups fat-free milk
1½ cups frozen light whipped topping, such as Cool Whip, thawed
2 cups hulled and halved fresh strawberries
2 cups fresh blueberries
2 cups fresh blackberries
2 tablespoons sugar substitute, such as DiabetiSweet or Splenda

Prepare the pound cake according to the recipe directions. Let cool completely, then cut half of the cake into 1½-inch cubes. Save the remaining cake for another use.

In a medium bowl, whisk the pudding mix into the milk until it begins to thicken, about 2 minutes. Fold in the whipped topping. Cover and refrigerate for 1 hour.

Meanwhile, in a large bowl, toss together the strawberries, blueberries, blackberries, and sugar substitute. Layer half of the cake cubes in the bottom of a clear trifle bowl. Top with a third of the berries, then half of the pudding. Repeat the layers of cake, berries, and pudding, topping with a final layer of berries.

Per Serving: 150 calories, 4 g protein, 21 g carbohydrate, 6 g fat, 1.5 g saturated fat, 20 mg cholesterol, 3 g dietary fiber, 120 mg sodium

Diet Exchanges: 1½ starches, 1 fat, or 1½ carbohydrate choices

Patti's Pumpkin Pie

Both the pie *lovers* and the pie *bakers* in my family are crazy about this pie, but not for the same reason. It's a favorite to the pie lovers for its taste (decadently delicious), while the pie bakers love it for its recipe (easy as, well, pie). When I was growing up, pumpkin pie was always made with granulated sugar and half-and-half by the great Southern cooks in my family. This healthier version uses sugar substitute and fat-free evaporated milk to keep the flavor without all of the calories.

Makes 8 servings

2 eggs
One 15-ounce can pumpkin
½ cup sugar substitute, such as DiabetiSweet
*   or Splenda*
1 teaspoon pumpkin pie spice
¼ teaspoon ground cinnamon
¼ teaspoon salt
One 12-ounce can fat-free evaporated milk
One 9-inch frozen piecrust or Perfect
*   Piecrust (page 192)*

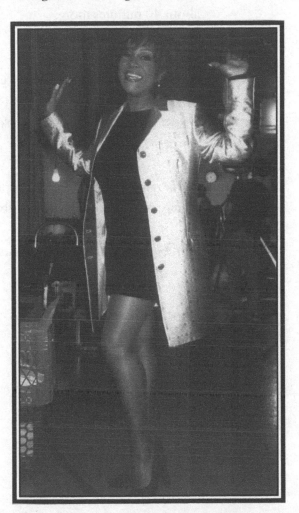

Hooray, hurrah, and hallelujah! With lighter desserts like this, I can fit into my old mini skirts.

Preheat the oven to 425°F.

In a medium bowl, whisk together the eggs, pumpkin, sugar substitute, pumpkin pie spice, cinnamon, salt, and evaporated milk. Pour into the piecrust.

Bake on a baking sheet for fifteen minutes. Reduce the oven temperature to 350°F and bake until a toothpick inserted in the center comes out almost clean, about 40 minutes more.

Patti's Pointers: Be sure that you use a sugar substitute that specifies that it can be used for cooking and baking. Many can't stand up to the heat! And before opening the can of evaporated milk, give it a quick shake to mix in the thickened milk that settles on the bottom of the can.

Per serving: 230 calories, 9 g protein, 28 g carbohydrate, 9 g fat, 3 g saturated fat, 60 mg cholesterol, 2 g dietary fiber, 310 mg sodium

Diet Exchanges: 2 starches, 2 fats, or 2 carbohydrate choices

Four-Flavor Sour Cream Pound Cake

Flavored with the tastes of vanilla, lemon, almond, and butter, you won't miss—or want—frosting!

Makes 16 servings

All-purpose flour, for dusting
2¼ cups cake flour
1½ teaspoons baking powder
½ teaspoon grated nutmeg (optional)
¼ teaspoon salt
½ cup margarine, softened
⅔ cup sugar substitute, such as DiabetiSweet or Splenda (see Patti's Pointers
  page 178)
7 tablespoons granulated sugar
1 teaspoon vanilla extract
1 teaspoon lemon extract
1 teaspoon almond extract
1 teaspoon butter-flavor extract
3 eggs, separated
1 cup reduced-fat sour cream

Preheat the oven to 350°F.

Coat a 9 × 5-inch nonstick loaf pan with fat-free cooking spray and dust with all-purpose flour.

In a medium bowl, combine the cake flour, baking powder, nutmeg (if using), and salt.

In a large bowl, using an electric mixer on medium speed, beat the margarine until light, about 30 seconds. Gradually beat in the sugar substitute and sugar until light and fluffy, about 3 minutes. Beat in the vanilla, lemon, almond, and butter flavor extracts. Beat in the egg yolks, one at a time, beating for 30 seconds after each addition.

Using a spoon, stir in the flour mixture alternately with the sour cream.

In a clean medium bowl, using clean beaters, beat the egg whites until soft peaks form when the beaters are lifted, about 5 minutes. Gently fold the egg whites into the batter. Spoon the batter into the prepared pan. Bake until a toothpick inserted in the center comes out clean, 55 to 65 minutes. Cool in the pan for 10 minutes. Invert onto a rack and cool completely.

Patti's Pointers: To get the highest volume from beaten egg whites, make sure that everything is clean and grease-free—the bowl, beaters, and scraper or spatula. Even a *tiny* speck of fat can keep the whites from increasing to their full volume.

Per Serving: 150 calories, 3 g protein, 17 g carbohydrate, 8 g fat, 2 g saturated fat, 30 mg cholesterol, 0 g dietary fiber, 130 mg sodium

Diet Exchanges: 1 starch, 1½ fats, or 1 carbohydrate choice

Chocolate Cream Pie

If you're a chocoholic, this is the recipe for you!

Makes 10 servings

15 sugar-free crème-filled chocolate sandwich cookies, crushed into crumbs
¼ cup margarine, melted
⅓ cup sugar substitute, such as DiabetiSweet or Splenda
¼ cup cornstarch
3 tablespoons unsweetened cocoa
2 cups fat-free half-and-half
1 teaspoon vanilla extract

In a medium bowl, mix together the cookie crumbs and melted margarine. Press the mixture in the bottom and up the sides of a 9-inch pie pan.

In a medium saucepan, whisk together the sugar substitute, cornstarch, and cocoa. Gradually whisk in the half-and-half over medium heat. Cook, whisking frequently, until the mixture is thickened to the texture of pudding, about 5 minutes. Whisk in the vanilla.

Pour the mixture into the prepared piecrust and let cool to room temperature. Cover and refrigerate for at least 4 hours, or up to 2 days.

Option: To make Chocolate Banana Cream Pie, line the bottom of the prepared piecrust with sliced bananas (about 1 large banana) before pouring in the chocolate pudding.

Patti's Pointers: An easy way to crush the cookies into crumbs is to put them in a Ziploc bag and pound them with a rolling pin. What a great stress reliever! And don't forget: A dollop of light whipped topping turns this creamy chocolate pie into a dreamy chocolate pie.

Per Serving: 120 calories, 3 g protein, 15 g carbohydrate, 6 g fat, 1 g saturated fat, 0 mg cholesterol, less than 1 g dietary fiber, 170 mg sodium

Diet Exchanges: 1 starch, 1 fat, or 1 carbohydrate choice

Awesome Apple Pie

Years of listening to the baking advice of my aunts Hattie Mae and Joshia Mae—
"For sweets you want dry, crisp surfaces, so bake uncovered; half-and-half won't
whip; if you must use something from a box or a bag, *puhleeze* doctor it up with
plenty of homemade touches"—make this pie truly awesome.

Makes 10 servings

*Two 9-inch frozen piecrusts or Perfect Piecrusts (page
192)*
*3 pounds Granny Smith apples, cored, peeled, and cut
into 1-inch pieces*
*¾ cup plus 1 teaspoon sugar substitute, such as Dia-
betiSweet or Splenda, divided (see Patti's Pointers
page 178)*
¼ cup all-purpose flour
½ teaspoon ground cinnamon
¼ teaspoon grated nutmeg
3 tablespoons egg substitute, such as Egg Beaters

Thaw one of the piecrusts, if frozen. Preheat the oven to
350°F.

In a large bowl, mix together the apples, ¾ cup sugar
substitute, the flour, cinnamon, and nutmeg.

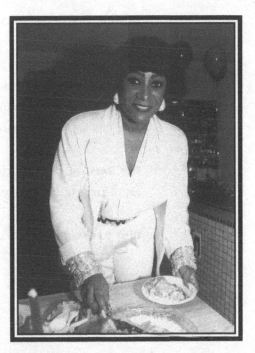

**Enjoying a piece of my Awesome Apple
Pie.**

Spoon into the frozen piecrust (filling will be mounded
up quite high).

Cut off and discard the rim of the thawed piecrust. On a floured surface, roll the
piecrust into an 11-inch circle. Cut the circle into strips, each about 1 inch wide.

Lay the strips over the apples in a lattice pattern (see Patti's Pointers below). Trim any overhang with kitchen scissors. Dab the edges of the dough with water and pinch onto the rim of the piecrust to seal.

Brush all of the exposed surfaces of dough with the egg substitute. Sprinkle with the remaining 1 teaspoon sugar substitute.

Bake on a baking sheet until the filling is bubbly and the crust is deep golden brown, about 1 hour and 15 minutes.

Option: If you like nuts, stir in ¼ cup chopped walnuts with the apples.

Patti's Pointers: To make a lattice top crust, cross the two longest strips of dough over the center of the pie. Cross the top strip with another long strip of dough. Fold back every other strip and lay the cross strips in place. Then put the folded-back strip in the original position.

Per Serving: 390 calories, 6 g protein, 59 g carbohydrate, 15 g fat, 4.5 g saturated fat, 5 mg cholesterol, 6 g dietary fiber, 180 mg sodium

Diet Exchanges: 3 starches, 3 fats, 1 fruit, or 4 carbohydrate choices

Old-fashioned Oatmeal Raisin Cookies

At my grocery store, you can find the fat-free fruit-based oil and shortening replacement right next to the Crisco. I like to use Smucker's because it measures one-for-one like shortening and, to me, it tastes a little better than some other brands.

Makes about 2 dozen cookies
Serving size is 1 cookie

¾ cup all-purpose flour
½ teaspoon baking soda
½ teaspoon ground cinnamon
¼ teaspoon salt
½ cup fat-free fruit-based oil and shortening replacement for baking
½ cup sugar substitute, such as DiabetiSweet or Splenda (see Patti's Pointers
    page 178)
¼ cup sugar-free brown sugar substitute, such as Brown Sugar Twin
¼ cup packed light brown sugar
1 egg
¼ cup fat-free milk
1 teaspoon vanilla extract
1½ cups old-fashioned oats
½ cup raisins
½ cup chopped walnuts, optional

Preheat the oven to 350°F.

In a small bowl, mix together the flour, baking soda, cinnamon, and salt.

In a large bowl, using an electric mixer, beat together the oil and shortening replacement, sugar substitute, brown sugar substitute, and brown sugar just until creamy, about 30 seconds. (When using fat-free fruit-based oil and shortening replacement, don't overbeat or your cookies will come out tough and chewy.) Beat in the egg, milk, and vanilla extract.

Stir in the flour mixture. Stir in the oats, raisins, and walnuts (if using).

Drop by well-rounded tablespoons onto ungreased cookie sheets, flattening the mounds slightly so the cookies will spread.

Bake until golden brown, about 10 minutes.

Patti's Pointers: I like to use Brown Sugar Twin spoonable brown sugar replacement. It can be used cup for cup like brown sugar, which makes it easier to use than other brands. And I think it tastes a little better, too.

Per Serving: 70 calories, 2 g protein, 12 g carbohydrate, 2 g fat, 0 g saturated fat, 10 mg cholesterol, less than 1 g dietary fiber, 55 mg sodium

Diet Exchanges: 1 starch, ½ fat, or 1 carbohydrate choice

No-Bake Cookies 'n' Cream Cheesecake

This is a great summer dessert because you don't have to turn on the oven! And when my hot flashes are giving me the blues, well, let's just say that's a blessing.

Makes 8 servings

CRUST

15 sugar-free crème-filled chocolate sandwich cookies, finely crushed
3 tablespoons margarine, melted

FILLING

One 8-ounce package reduced-fat cream cheese, softened
One 8-ounce package fat-free cream cheese, softened
⅓ cup sugar substitute, such as DiabetiSweet or Splenda
½ teaspoon vanilla extract
13 sugar-free crème-filled chocolate sandwich cookies
One 8-ounce tub frozen light whipped topping, such as Cool Whip, thawed

To make the crust: In a medium bowl, combine the 15 crushed cookies and margarine. Press the mixture into the bottom and up the sides of a 9-inch pie pan.

To make the filling: In a large bowl, using an electric mixer on medium speed, beat the cream cheese, sugar substitute, and vanilla extract until creamy, about 1 minute.

Coarsely crush 10 of the cookies and stir into the cream cheese mixture. Fold in 2 cups of the whipped topping. Spoon into the prepared piecrust, cover with foil, and refrigerate for 2 hours before serving.

Spread the remaining whipped topping over the pie. Arrange the remaining 3 cookies in the center of the pie for garnish.

Per Serving: 340 calories, 8 g protein, 29 g carbohydrate, 21 g fat, 8 g saturated fat, 29 mg cholesterol, less than 1 g dietary fiber, 460 mg sodium

Diet Exchanges: 2 starches, 4 fats, or 2 carbohydrate choices

Decadently Delicious Chocolate Mousse

For an oh-so-cute presentation, serve this simple and delicious dessert in martini glasses!

Makes 4 servings

1½ cups fat-free half-and-half
One 1.4-ounce package fat-free, sugar-free instant
* chocolate pudding mix*
One 8-ounce tub frozen light whipped topping, such as
* Cool Whip, thawed*

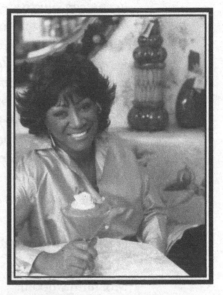

In a large bowl, whisk together the half-and-half and pudding mix until creamy, about 2 minutes.

Fold in the whipped topping, reserving ¼ cup of it for decoration.

Divide the mousse evenly among individual dessert bowls and refrigerate for 20 minutes, or up to 2 days.

Using the reserved 2 tablespoons of whipped topping, dollop ½ tablespoon on each serving.

See how cute the mousse looks in a martini glass? (Photo by Ernest Washington)

Patti's Pointers: To take this dessert over the rainbow, stir in ½ teaspoon rum extract along with the half-and-half.

Per Serving: 70 calories, 2 g protein, 9 g carbohydrate, 3 g fat, 0 g saturated fat, 0 mg cholesterol, 0 g dietary fiber, 170 mg sodium

Diet Exchanges: ½ starch, ½ fat, or ½ carbohydrate choice

Blue Ribbon Blueberry Pie

Makes 10 servings

½ cup sugar substitute, such as DiabetiSweet or Splenda (see Patti's Pointers
 page 178)
¼ cup granulated sugar
¼ cup all-purpose flour, divided
¼ cup egg substitute, such as Egg Beaters
⅔ cup fat-free sour cream
¼ teaspoon vanilla extract
¼ teaspoon butter-flavor extract
2 cups fresh or frozen blueberries
One 9-inch frozen piecrust or Perfect Piecrust (page 192)
2 tablespoons sugar-free brown sugar replacement, such as Brown Sugar Twin
2 tablespoons chopped walnuts
1 tablespoon margarine, softened

Preheat the oven to 400°F.

In a large bowl, stir together the sugar substitute, granulated sugar, 2 tablespoons
of the flour, the egg substitute, sour cream, and vanilla and butter-flavor extracts.
Mix until smooth.

Stir in the blueberries and pour into the piecrust.

Bake on a baking sheet until the filling just starts to bubble, about 25 minutes.

In a cup, using a fork, mix together the remaining 2 tablespoons flour, the brown
sugar replacement, walnuts, and margarine. Break into fine crumbs and sprinkle
over the pie. Bake until the filling is bubbly and the topping is golden brown,
about 10 minutes more.

Option: If you use frozen blueberries for this recipe, you'll need two 12-ounce bags.

Per Serving: 210 calories, 6 g protein, 30 g carbohydrate, 8 g fat, 1.5 g saturated fat, 0 mg cholesterol, 1 g dietary fiber, 190 mg sodium

Diet Exchanges: 2 starches, 1½ fats, or 2 carbohydrate choices

Perfect Piecrust

Sometimes, not often but sometimes, only a homemade piecrust will do. Most times, however, it's best (and so much easier!) to use frozen piecrust. That's because commercial machines can roll a piecrust much thinner than human hands ever could, I don't care how skilled a baker a person may be. And the thinner the piecrust, the lower it is in fat and calories. Don't tell Aunt Hattie or Aunt Josh, but since I learned I was diabetic, I bake almost all my pies with frozen crusts. That's why I had to go on a serious search for a great, yet light, homemade one. Cookbook author and recipe developer David Joachim shared this one with me. I tasted lots of others but his was the hands-down winner.

Makes 8 servings

1½ cups all-purpose flour
½ teaspoon salt
¼ cup cold butter-flavored vegetable shortening
¼ cup cold reduced-fat cream cheese
2 teaspoons lemon juice
¼ cup ice water

In a large bowl, combine the flour and salt. Using a pastry blender or fork, quickly cut in the shortening and cream cheese until the mixture resembles coarse meal.

In a cup, combine the lemon juice and 2 tablespoons of the ice water. Mix into the dough just until moist. Mix in just enough remaining ice water so that the dough can be shaped into a ball. Gather the dough into a ball and flatten it into a disk in the bowl. Cover and refrigerate for 1 hour, or up to 8 hours.

Preheat the oven to 400°F.

Roll the dough between sheets of lightly floured waxed or parchment paper, into a 12-inch circle. Remove the top sheet and carefully invert the dough into the center of a 9-inch pie pan. Remove the remaining sheet of paper and carefully fit the dough into the pan without stretching it.

Crimp the edges with your fingers or a fork and prick the bottom of the crust with a fork to prevent bubbling.

Line the inside of the crust with heavy foil. Bake on a baking sheet for 7 minutes.

Remove the foil and bake until lightly golden, about 7 minutes more. Cool on a rack.

Option: To make a Perfect Nut Crust, stir 2 tablespoons finely ground almonds or walnuts into the flour and salt.

Patti's Pointers: There are two secrets to a tender, flaky piecrust. The first is to handle the dough as little as possible. The second is to keep everything cold. Especially the fat. Cold fat in a hot oven creates steam, which puffs apart the layers in the crust and makes flaky pastry. If the fat warms up before it gets to the oven, it melts and gets absorbed by the flour, creating a tough crust. If you make a pie dough on a hot day, chill all your ingredients and equipment in the refrigerator. If the dough warms up and gets sticky as you work, pop it back in the fridge for 20 minutes before continuing.

Per Serving: 160 calories, 3 g protein, 19 g carbohydrate, 8 g fat, 2.5 g saturated fat, 5 mg cholesterol, less than 1 g dietary fiber, 25 mg sodium

Diet Exchanges: 1 starch, 1½ fats, or 1 carbohydrate choice

Layered Banana Pudding

Fat-free milk and sugar-free vanilla wafers turn this classic dessert into one everyone in the family can enjoy.

Makes 12 servings

Two 1-ounce boxes fat-free, sugar-free instant vanilla pudding mix
1 cup reduced-fat sour cream
One 8-ounce tub frozen light whipped topping, such as Cool Whip, thawed
3 cups fat-free milk
Two 5.5-ounce boxes sugar-free Nilla Wafers
4 ripe bananas, sliced
1 teaspoon ground cinnamon
1 teaspoon sugar substitute, such as DiabetiSweet or Splenda

In a large bowl, using an electric mixer on low speed, beat together the pudding mix, sour cream, whipped topping, and milk until creamy, about 2 minutes.

Arrange a layer of Nilla Wafers on the bottom of a 13 × 9-inch rectangular pan, using a little less than half of the cookies. Set aside 12 cookies for decorating the top.

Layer half of the banana slices on top of the wafers in the pan. Pour half of the pudding over the bananas.

In a small bowl, mix together the cinnamon and sugar substitute. Sprinkle half of the cinnamon-sugar over the pudding. Repeat the layers, using the remaining cookies, sliced bananas, pudding, and cinnamon-sugar.

Decorate the top with the 12 reserved cookies. Cover with foil and refrigerate for at least 2 hours, or up to 1 day, before serving.

Patti's Pointers: Be sure to use the sugar-free version of round Nilla Wafers in this recipe. They look so cute—like little buttons—decorating the top of this crowd-pleasing dessert.

Per Serving: 270 calories, 4 g protein, 40 g carbohydrate, 14 g fat, 7 g saturated fat, 10 mg cholesterol, 1 g dietary fiber, 390 mg sodium

Diet Exchanges: 2 starches, 2 fruits, 3 fats, or 2½ carbohydrate choices

Spectacular Spice Cake

Makes 16 servings

2 cups cake flour
1 teaspoon baking powder
1 teaspoon cinnamon
½ teaspoon ground nutmeg
½ teaspoon ground ginger
¼ teaspoon salt
½ cup margarine, softened
1 cup sugar substitute such as DiabetiSweet or Splenda (see Patti's Pointers
   page 178)
⅔ cup brown sugar substitute, such as Brown Sugar Twin
⅓ cup packed light brown sugar
3 eggs, separated
1 teaspoon vanilla extract
1 cup 1 percent low-fat buttermilk
1 cup raisins
1 cup chopped toasted walnuts

Preheat the oven to 350°F. Coat a 9-cup or 10-cup tube pan with fat-free cooking spray.

In a medium bowl, whisk together the flour, baking powder, cinnamon, nutmeg, ginger, and salt.

In a large bowl, using an electric mixer on medium speed, beat the margarine until light, about 1 minute. Beat in the sugar substitute, brown sugar substitute, and brown sugar until fluffy, about 3 minutes. Add the egg yolks, one at a time, beating for 30 seconds after each addition. Beat in the vanilla.

Beat in the flour mixture alternating with the buttermilk and beating for 30 seconds after each addition.

In a clean medium bowl, using clean beaters, beat the egg whites until soft peaks form when the beaters are lifted, about 5 minutes. Fold into the batter. Fold in the raisins and walnuts.

Scrape into the prepared pan and bake until a toothpick inserted in the center comes out clean, 20 to 30 minutes. Cool in the pan for 10 minutes. Invert onto a rack and cool completely.

Option: This ring cake looks fabulous with a glaze (low-sugar of course!). In a medium bowl, melt 1½ tablespoons reduced-calorie margarine in the microwave oven, about 30 seconds on medium. Whisk in 1½ tablespoons fat-free half-and-half and ¾ teaspoon vanilla extract. Then whisk in ¾ cup sugar substitute and ⅓ cup powdered sugar. Drizzle evenly over the cooled cake.

Patti's Pointers: I like to toast nuts before using them. It coaxes out every bit of their flavor. While the oven is preheating, spread the nuts on a baking sheet and bake until fragrant and toasty, about 5 minutes. Watch carefully so they don't burn!

Per Serving: 210 calories, 5 g protein, 24 g carbohydrate, 11 g fat, 1.5 g saturated fat, 40 mg cholesterol, 1 g dietary fiber, 170 mg sodium

Diet Exchanges: 1½ starches, 2 fats, or 1½ carbohydrate choices

Strawberry Ice Cream Pie
with Chocolate Crust

The name says it all, right?

Makes 10 servings

3 tablespoons margarine, melted
15 sugar-free crème-filled chocolate sandwich cookies, crushed
2 pints (4 cups) no-sugar-added strawberry ice cream
1½ cups fresh strawberries, top removed

Place the margarine in a medium bowl. Microwave on medium heat until melted, 30 to 45 seconds. Stir in the crushed cookies until well blended.

Press the mixture firmly into the bottom and up the sides of a 9-inch pie pan.

Place the ice cream in a large bowl and let soften for 15 minutes.

Meanwhile, cut ½ cup of the strawberries into quarters and add to the bowl. Stir together the strawberries and ice cream.

Spoon the ice cream mixture evenly into the pie crust. Cover tightly with foil and freeze for at least 6 hours, or up to 3 days.

Before serving, slice the remaining 1 cup strawberries and arrange decoratively over the pie. Re-cover with the foil and let soften in the refrigerator for 45 minutes.

Patti's Pointers: My favorite brand of no-sugar-added strawberry ice cream is Edy's Grand. If you can't find it in your supermarket, experiment with different brands until you find your favorite.

Per Serving: 180 calories, 4 g protein, 26 g carbohydrate, 7 g fat, 2 g saturated fat, 5 mg cholesterol, 2 g dietary fiber, 180 mg sodium

Diet Exchanges: 1 starch, 1 fruit, or 2 carbohydrate choices

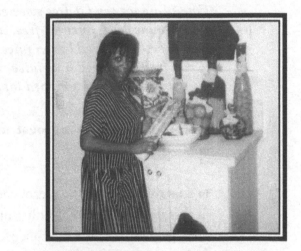

Preparing a big green salad for dinner so I can have strawberry ice cream pie for dessert.

Smooth-as-Silk Lemon-Lime Pie

For a drop-dead presentation, arrange a few thin, halved slices of lemon and lime in the center of the pie before serving.

Makes 10 servings

One 9-inch frozen pie shell or baked Perfect Piecrust (page 192)
One 8-ounce package reduced-fat cream cheese, softened
One 14-ounce can fat-free sweetened condensed milk
One 8-ounce container fat-free, sugar-free light lemon-flavor yogurt
¼ cup fresh-squeezed lemon juice
¼ cup fresh-squeezed lime juice
1½ cups frozen light whipped topping, such as Cool Whip, thawed

Prepare the baked pastry crust according to package or recipe instructions. Let cool.

In a large bowl, beat the cream cheese until light and fluffy, about 1 minute. Beat in the condensed milk, beating until smooth, about 30 seconds. Beat in the yogurt, lemon juice, and lime juice.

Fold in the whipped topping. Scrape into the prepared piecrust (filling will be mounded quite high).

Refrigerate for at least 4 hours or up to 1 day.

Per serving: 320 calories, 10 g protein, 44 g carbohydrate, 12 g fat, 4.5 g saturated fat, 20 mg cholesterol, less than 1 g dietary fiber, 260 mg sodium

Diet Exchanges: 3 starches, 2 fats, or 3 carbohydrate choices

Peach Upside-down Cake

I like to use an 8-inch cast-iron skillet when I make this cake. It reminds me of the way Chubby used to make hers. If your skillet doesn't have ovenproof (metal) handles, you can still use it. Just wrap the handle in several layers of heavy-duty foil to protect it in the oven.

Makes 10 servings

2 tablespoons packed light brown sugar
2 tablespoons brown sugar substitute, such as Brown Sugar Twin
¾ cup sugar substitute, such as DiabetiSweet or Splenda, divided (see Patti's Pointers page 178)
2 tablespoons plus ⅓ cup margarine
2 ripe peaches, peeled, pitted, and sliced (about 2 cups)
½ teaspoon grated nutmeg
1½ cups cake flour
½ teaspoon baking powder
¼ teaspoon salt
3 tablespoons sugar
1 egg
1 teaspoon vanilla extract
1 teaspoon butter-flavor extract
½ cup fat-free half-and-half

Preheat the oven to 350°F.

In a small bowl, stir together the brown sugar, brown sugar substitute, and ¼ cup of the sugar substitute.

In an 8-inch or 10-inch ovenproof skillet, melt 2 tablespoons of the margarine. Sprinkle evenly with the sugar mixture.

Arrange the peach slices in the pan in overlapping concentric circles starting from the center. Sprinkle with the nutmeg.

In a medium bowl, combine the flour, baking powder, and salt.

In a large bowl, beat the remaining ⅓ cup margarine until light, about 30 seconds. Beat in the sugar and remaining ½ cup sugar substitute until light and fluffy, about 30 seconds.

Beat in the egg, vanilla extract, and butter-flavor extract.

Beat in the flour mixture alternately with the half-and-half, beating for 30 seconds after each addition. Spoon the batter over the peaches.

Bake until lightly golden and a toothpick inserted into the center of the cake comes out clean, 30 to 35 minutes. Invert onto a serving plate and replace any topping that may have fallen off.

Option: If you can't find fresh peaches, you can use two 15-ounce cans sliced light freestone peaches in extra light syrup, drained.

Patti's Pointers: To peel fresh peaches, bring a pot of water to boil over high heat. Drop in the peaches to shock them for 30 to 45 seconds. Transfer with a slotted spoon to a bowl of ice water to shock them again. After all that shocking, the peels will slip right off! If a peach has a tough skin, use a paring knife to peel it away.

Per Serving: 110 calories, 2 g protein, 21 g carbohydrate, 2.5 g fat, 0 g saturated fat, 0 mg cholesterol, less than 1 g dietary fiber, 120 mg sodium

Diet Exchanges: 1½ starches, ½ fat, or 1½ carbohydrate choices

Melt-in-Your-Mouth
Chocolate Chip Cookies

Makes about 2 dozen cookies

Serving size is 1 cookie

1¾ cups all-purpose flour
1 teaspoon baking soda
¼ teaspoon salt
½ cup margarine, softened
¾ cup sugar substitute, such as DiabetiSweet or Splenda (see Patti's Pointers
   page 178)
¼ cup sugar-free brown sugar substitute, such as Brown Sugar Twin
½ cup brown sugar
1 egg
2 teaspoons vanilla extract
1 cup (6 ounces) semisweet chocolate chips

Preheat the oven to 375°F.

In a small bowl, whisk together the flour, baking soda, and salt.

In a large bowl, using an electric mixer on medium speed, beat the margarine
until light, about 1 minute. Beat in the sugar substitute, brown sugar substitute,
brown sugar, egg, and vanilla extract. Beat until fluffy.

Stir in the flour mixture.

Stir in the chocolate chips.

Drop the dough by well-rounded tablespoons onto ungreased cookie sheets, flattening the mounds slightly so they will spread.

Bake until lightly golden, 8 to 10 minutes. Cool on the baking sheet for 5 minutes. Transfer to racks to cool completely.

Patti's Pointers: Be careful not to overbake these cookies. A little underdone and moist inside tastes better than a little overdone and dry inside.

Per Serving: 120 calories, 2 g protein, 16 g carbohydrate, 6 g fat, 2 g saturated fat, 10 mg cholesterol, less than 1 g dietary fiber, 135 mg sodium

Diet Exchanges: 1 starch, 1 fat, or 1 carbohydrate choice

Killer Chocolate Cake
with Guilt-free Glaze

Makes 10 servings

CAKE

⅓ cup margarine
¼ cup unsweetened cocoa powder
½ cup water
¾ cup sugar substitute, such as DiabetiSweet or Splenda (see Patti's Pointers
    page 178)
¼ cup packed light brown sugar
1 egg
⅓ cup 1 percent low-fat buttermilk
1 teaspoon vanilla extract
1 teaspoon butter-flavor extract
1 teaspoon chocolate-flavor extract (optional)
1 cup cake flour
½ teaspoon baking soda

GLAZE

1 tablespoon reduced-calorie margarine
1 tablespoon fat-free half-and-half
½ teaspoon vanilla extract
2 tablespoons unsweetened cocoa powder
½ cup sugar substitute, such as DiabetiSweet or Splenda
¼ cup powdered sugar

To make the cake: Preheat the oven to 350°F. Coat an 8-inch cake pan with fat-free cooking spray.

In a medium saucepan over high heat, whisk together the margarine, cocoa powder, and water. Bring to a boil, stirring often.

Remove from the heat and whisk in the sugar substitute, brown sugar, egg, buttermilk, vanilla extract, butter-flavor extract, chocolate-flavor extract (if using), flour, and baking soda. Whisk vigorously for 2 minutes.

Pour the batter into the prepared pan. Bake until a toothpick inserted in the center comes out clean, 30 to 40 minutes. Cool in the pan for 10 minutes. Invert onto a rack and cool completely. When cool, transfer to a serving plate.

To make the glaze: Place the margarine in a small microwaveable bowl. Microwave on medium heat until melted, about 30 seconds. Whisk in the half-and-half, vanilla extract, unsweetened cocoa powder, sugar substitute, and powdered sugar. Spread evenly over the top and sides of the cooled cake.

Per Serving: 130 calories, 2 g protein, 14 g carbohydrate, 7 g fat, 1.5 g saturated fat, 20 mg cholesterol, less than 1 g dietary fiber, 160 mg sodium

Diet Exchanges: 1 starch, 1 fat, or 1 carbohydrate choice

Chocolate Pecan Pie

Makes 10 servings

¼ cup margarine
⅓ cup unsweetened cocoa powder
1 pint (2 cups) fat-free half-and-half
1 tablespoon brown sugar substitute, such as Brown Sugar Twin
1 tablespoon packed light brown sugar
2 eggs, beaten
2 egg whites
½ teaspoon vanilla extract
1 teaspoon chocolate-flavor extract
⅓ cup chopped toasted pecans
One 9-inch frozen pie shell or Perfect Piecrust (page 192)

Preheat the oven to 350°F.

Melt the margarine in a medium saucepan over medium-low heat. Whisk in the cocoa powder until smooth. Gradually whisk in the half-and-half, brown sugar substitute, brown sugar, eggs, and egg whites. Remove from the heat and stir in the vanilla extract, chocolate-flavor extract, and pecans.

Place the piecrust on a baking sheet. Pour in the chocolate filling and bake until set and a toothpick inserted in the center comes out clean, 40 to 45 minutes.

Patti's Pointers: To toast the pecans, spread them on a baking sheet and bake while the oven is preheating until fragrant and toasty, about 5 minutes.

Per Serving: 250 calories, 7 g protein, 21 g carbohydrate, 16 g fat, 3.5 g saturated fat, 45 mg cholesterol, 2 g dietary fiber, 230 mg sodium

Diet Exchanges: 1½ starches, 3 fats, or 1½ carbohydrate choices

Child, That's Good Chocolate Tapioca

Thanks to quick-cooking tapioca, you can make this dessert in minutes. But tell everybody it took you all day. ⤺

Makes 10 servings

3 cups fat-free half-and-half
3 tablespoons sugar substitute, such as DiabetiSweet or Splenda
¼ cup unsweetened cocoa powder
¼ cup quick-cooking tapioca
¼ teaspoon salt
1 teaspoon margarine, melted
1 teaspoon vanilla extract
1 teaspoon butter-flavor extract

Pour the half-and-half into a medium saucepan and bring to a simmer over medium heat. Whisk in the sugar substitute, cocoa powder, tapioca, and salt. Cook and stir until soft, about 2 minutes.

Whisk in the margarine, vanilla extract, and butter-flavor extract.

Pour the mixture into a large serving bowl. Cover with foil and refrigerate for at least 3 hours, or up to 2 days.

Per Serving: 90 calories, 5 g protein, 14 g carbohydrate, 0.5 g fat, 0 g saturated fat, 5 mg cholesterol, less than 1 g dietary fiber, 150 mg sodium

Diet Exchanges: 1 starch or 1 carbohydrate choice

Buttermilk Chocolate Almond Cake

The ground almonds in this cake boost the nutty flavor and enrich the texture of the cake. But if you don't have a food processor, you can skip them. The cake will work fine without them.

Makes 16 servings

⅓ cup almonds
1¼ cups sugar substitute, such as DiabetiSweet or Splenda, divided (see Patti's Pointers page 178)
2 cups cake flour
¾ cup unsweetened cocoa powder
2 teaspoons baking soda
1 teaspoon salt
1½ cups 1 percent low-fat buttermilk
½ cup vegetable oil
¼ cup fat-free fruit-based butter and oil replacement
2 eggs
2 egg whites
¼ cup packed light brown sugar
2 teaspoons almond-flavor extract

Preheat the oven to 350°F. Coat a 10-cup nonstick tube pan with fat-free cooking spray.

In a food processor, process the almonds with 1 tablespoon of the sugar substitute using short pulses until the almonds are finely ground. Transfer to a large bowl. Whisk in the flour, cocoa powder, baking soda, and salt.

In another large bowl, whisk together the buttermilk, oil, fat-free fruit-based butter and oil replacement, eggs, egg whites, remaining 1 cup plus 3 tablespoons sugar substitute, brown sugar, and almond-flavor extract. Whisk until well blended. Stir in the flour mixture.

Scrape the batter into the prepared pan. Bake until a toothpick inserted in the center comes out clean, 30 to 40 minutes. Cool in the pan for 10 minutes. Invert onto a rack and cool completely.

Option: To take this cake to the next level, drizzle the cooled cake with a double recipe of Guilt-Free Glaze (page 205), then decorate with sliced almonds.

Per Serving: 170 calories, 4 g protein, 17 g carbohydrate, 10 g fat, 1.5 g saturated fat, 25 mg cholesterol, 2 g dietary fiber, 340 mg sodium

Diet Exchanges: 1 starch, 2 fats, or 1 carbohydrate choice

Blueberry Cake

Makes 14 servings

2 cups cake flour
1 teaspoon baking powder
¼ teaspoon salt
1½ cups fresh blueberries
4 tablespoons margarine, softened
1¼ cups sugar substitute, such as DiabetiSweet or Splenda (see Patti's Pointers page 178)
¼ cup granulated sugar
2 eggs, separated
1 teaspoon lemon extract
1 teaspoon butter-flavor extract
1 cup 1 percent low-fat buttermilk

Preheat the oven to 350°F. Coat a 9-cup or 10-cup nonstick tube pan with fat-free cooking spray.

In a medium bowl, whisk together the flour, baking powder, and salt.

Transfer ½ cup of the flour mixture to another medium bowl. Add the blueberries and toss to coat with flour mixture. Set aside.

In a large bowl, using an electric mixer on medium speed, beat the margarine until light, about 1 minute. Beat in the sugar substitute and sugar until fluffy, 1 minute.

Beat in the egg yolks, one at a time, beating for 30 seconds after each addition. Beat in the lemon extract and butter-flavor extract.

Beat in the flour mixture, alternating with the buttermilk, beating for 30 seconds after each addition.

In a clean medium bowl, using clean beaters, beat the egg whites until soft peaks form when the beaters are lifted, about 5 minutes. Fold into the batter.

Fold in the blueberries.

Scrape into the prepared pan and bake until a toothpick inserted in the center comes out clean, 35 to 40 minutes. Cool in the pan for 10 minutes. Invert onto a rack and cool completely.

Option: This wonderful ring cake is over-the-top with a simple lemon glaze. In a medium bowl, melt 1½ tablespoons reduced-calorie margarine in the microwave oven, about 30 seconds on medium. Whisk in 1½ tablespoons fat-free half-and-half and 1 teaspoon lemon juice. Then whisk in ¾ cup sugar substitute, such as DiabetiSweet or Splenda, and ⅓ cup powdered sugar. Drizzle evenly over the cooled cake. Garnish with grated lemon peel if you really want to impress.

Per Serving: 120 calories, 3 g protein, 18 g carbohydrate, 4.5 g fat, 1 g saturated fat, 35 mg cholesterol, less than 1 g dietary fiber, 150 mg sodium

Diet Exchanges: 1 starch, 1 fat, or 1 carbohydrate choice

Beyond Good Black Forest Parfaits

These are almost as cute as the Very Berry Trifle! (page 176)

Makes 8 servings

One 4-ounce package reduced-fat cream cheese, softened
One 4-ounce package fat-free cream cheese, softened
1¼ cups fat-free half-and-half
One 1.4-ounce package sugar-free, fat-free chocolate instant pudding mix
5 sugar-free crème-filled chocolate sandwich cookies, crushed (about ½ cup)
One 21-ounce can cherry pie filling

In a medium bowl, using an electric mixer, beat the cream cheese until light and fluffy, about 1 minute. Beat in ½ cup of the half-and-half until smooth, about 1 minute. Beat in the pudding mix and remaining ¾ cup of half-and-half.

Spoon half of the pudding mixture into dessert cups or small parfait glasses. Sprinkle the cookie crumbs over the pudding.

Set aside ½ cup of the cherry pie filling. Divide the remaining cherry pie filling among the cups, spooning over the cookie crumbs. Spoon the remaining pudding mixture over the cherry pie filling. Garnish each dessert cup or small parfait glass with the reserved ½ cup cherry pie filling.

Cover with foil and refrigerate for at least 1 hour, or up to 2 days.

Option: These parfaits scream for a dollop of light whipped topping. Give it to them!

Per Serving: 180 calories, 6 g protein, 32 g carbohydrate, 3.5 g fat, 2 g saturated fat, 10 mg cholesterol, less than 1 g dietary fiber, 330 mg sodium

Diet Exchanges: 2 starches, ½ fat, or 2 carbohydrate choices

Best Ever Brownies

When you smell these brownies baking, you'll be tempted to eat them the minute they come out of the oven, but don't! It's actually better to let them cool first. Hot brownies are hard to cut neatly, and if you do cut them, steam escapes, releasing moisture and making the brownies dry. And I don't know about you but I'm not hardly trying to use my calories on a dried-up brownie. If warm brownies are your weakness, reheat them briefly in a 350°F oven or for 15 seconds in a microwave oven.

Makes 16 brownies

Serving size is 1 brownie

¾ cup flour
½ teaspoon baking powder
½ teaspoon salt
¾ cup sugar substitute, such as DiabetiSweet or Splenda (see Patti's Pointers
    page 178)
⅓ cup sugar
3 eggs
1 tablespoon vanilla extract
¼ cup margarine
¼ cup chocolate chips
⅔ cup unsweetened cocoa powder
¼ cup fat-free fruit-based butter and oil replacement
1 teaspoon instant espresso powder (optional)
½ cup chopped toasted walnuts

Preheat the oven to 350°F. Line an 8-inch-square baking pan with foil and coat the foil with fat-free cooking spray.

In a small bowl, whisk together the flour, baking powder, and salt.

In a large bowl, whisk together the sugar substitute, sugar, eggs, and vanilla.

In a medium microwave-safe bowl, combine the margarine and chocolate chips, and microwave on medium heat just until melted, about 30 seconds. Whisk in the cocoa powder, fat-free fruit-based butter and oil replacement, and instant espresso (if using). Stir into the sugar mixture. Stir in the flour mixture and walnuts.

Scrape into the prepared pan and bake until a toothpick inserted into the center comes out with moist crumbs on it, 25 to 30 minutes. Cool in the pan for 5 minutes. Using the foil, lift the brownies out of the pan and cool completely on a rack. Cut into 16 pieces.

Patti's Pointers: Don't you just hate it when you can't get all of the brownies out of the pan? Well, the foil "sling" in this recipe solves that all too common problem. By lining the pan with foil, you can just lift the whole cake of brownies out of the pan, cool them, then cut them easily. Don't you just love it when a plan comes together?

Per Serving: 120 calories, 3 g protein, 14 g carbohydrate, 7 g fat, 1.5 g saturated fat, 25 mg cholesterol, 2 g dietary fiber, 135 mg sodium

Diet Exchanges: 1 starch, 1 fat, or 1 carbohydrate choice

Index

K

Killer Chocolate Cake with Guilt-Free
Glaze, 205–206

L

Lamb Chops LaBelle, 91–92
Layered Banana Pudding, 194–195
Lemon
    Hellacious Halibut with Lemon
        and Cilantro, 74–75
    Lemon-Basil Chicken Pitas, 30
    Smooth-as-Silk Lemon-Lime Pie,
        200
Lemon-Basil Chicken Pitas, 30
Lime, in Smooth-as-Silk Lemon-Lime
    Pie, 200
Llona's Steak Sandwiches, 25–27
Lobster
    Daniel's Chilled Spring Carrot
        Soup with Lobster and Lime,
        19–21
    Lucious Lobster Salad, 9–10
Luther's Italian Chicken Soup, 14–16

M

Magnificent Monkfish with
    Caramelized Onions and
    Olives, 55–56
Mahimahi, in Sublime Seafood Grill,
    51–52
Mango Salsa, Good-as-It-Gets Grilled
    Chicken with, 127–128

Marvelous Minted Snap Peas, 162
Meat dishes. *See also* Chicken; Turkey
    "Barbecue" Pork Chops, 101–102
    Burnin' Beef Stroganoff, 93–94
    Down-Home Pork Chops in
        Guilt-Free Gravy, 95–96
    Lamb Chops LaBelle, 91–92
    Melt-in-Your-Mouth Roast Ten-
        derloin, 88–89
    Pass-It-On Pork Crown Roast,
        104–106
    Patti's Potato and Ham Frittata,
        97–98
    For Real Veal Meat Loaf, 84–85
    Righteous Rump Roast, 99–100
    Seven-Layer Beef Skillet, 82–83
    Sooo Good Swiss Steak, 86–87
    Veal Parmigiana, 78–79
    Verrrry Good Veal Chops with
        Mushroom Gravy, 80–81
Melt-in-Your-Mouth Chocolate Chip
    Cookies, 203–204
Melt-in-Your-Mouth Roast Tenderloin,
    88–89
Mint, in Marvelous Minted Snap Peas,
    162
Monkfish, Magnificent, with
    Caramelized Onions and
    Olives, 55–56
Mousse, Decadently Delicious Choco-
    late, 189
Mushrooms
    Fabulous French Onion and
        Mushroom Turkey Burgers,
        31–32
    Heavenly Herb-baked Chicken
        and Mushroom Casserole,
        143–144